Understanding X-Rays:
A Plain English Approach

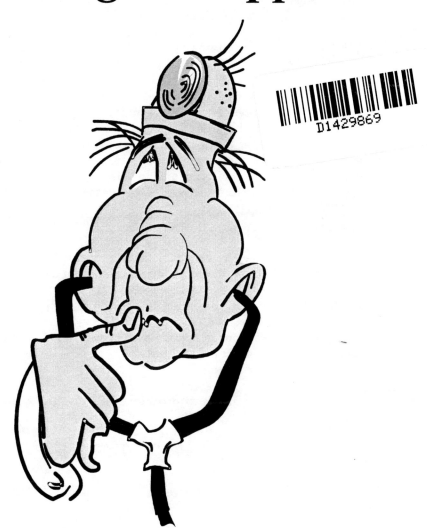

Mikel A. Rothenberg, M.D.

"This publication is designed to provide general information prepared by professionals in regard to subject matter covered. It is sold with the understanding that the publisher is not engaged in rendering legal, accounting, or other professional service. Although prepared by professionals, this publication should not be utilized as a substitute for professional service in specific situations. If legal advice or other expert assistance is required, the service of a professional should be sought."

From a Declaration of Principles jointly adopted by a Committee of the American Bar Association and a Committee of Publishers.

Opinions expressed by program faculty members do not necessarily reflect the opinions of this company, its management or employees.

PESI publications are designed to provide accurate information with regard to the subject matter covered. Attorneys and other professionals using PESI publications in dealing with specific legal matters should also research original sources of authority.

For information on this and other PESI manuals, audiocassettes and videotapes, please call

800-843-7763

Visit our web site at www.pesi.com

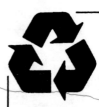

recycled paper

Every year Professional Education Systems, Inc., produces more than 45,000 seminar manuals. To help protect our environment, we have chosen to use recycled paper, reduce the size of our manuals, and recycle all materials at our home office. Our efforts were recognized on Earth Day in the April 19, 1991 issue (p. 2B) of *USA Today*:
"Professional Education Systems doesn't make money from recycling; it donates waste paper to a nonprofit recycler."

For the past eight years and in the future, PESI is committed to doing our part to help save the environment — **together, we will make a difference.**

We welcome your comments. Please call our Customer Service Department at 800-843-7763.

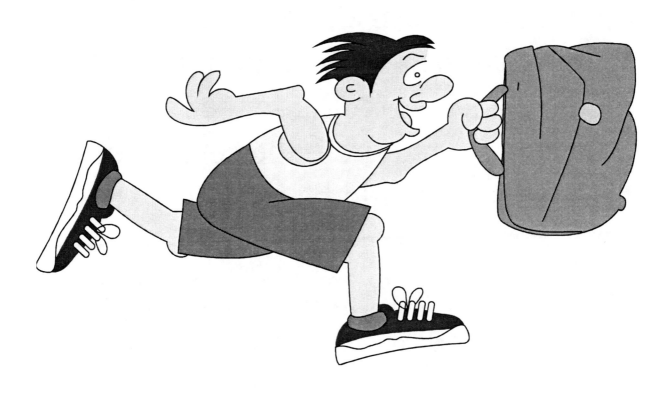

DISCLAIMER — This publication is designed to provide general information prepared by professionals about x-rays. It is sold with the understanding that the publisher and the author are not engaged in rendering medical, legal, accounting, or other professional service. Although prepared by professionals, this publication should not be used as a substitute for the expert opinion of a licensed medical radiologist in specific situations. If medical advice or other expert assistance is required, the service of a professional should be sought.

Modified from a Declaration of Principles jointly adopted by a Committee of the American Bar Association and a Committee of Publishers.

MATERIALS PROVIDED BY

Mikel A. Rothenberg, MD, is a board-certified internal medicine specialist with a special interest in critical care and emergency medicine. He has served as an ICU/CCU director as well as physician advisor for both air and ground ambulance services. Dr. Rothenberg has written four books: *Advanced Medical Life Support: Adult Medical Emergencies*; *Emergency Department Standards of Care: A Lawyer's Guide*; the Barron's *Dictionary of Medical Terms*; and *Anatomy and Physiology for Lawyers*. He is also the executive editor of an advanced cardiac life support update newsletter, *ACLS Alert*; and the author of "Life Disc," a computerized ACLS review program, and many articles for prehospital care journals. In addition to working as an emergency educator and medicolegal expert in Cleveland, Ohio, Dr. Rothenberg travels internationally presenting courses on ACLS, adult medical emergencies, laboratory testing and medical negligence. He is a recipient of PESI's Excellence in Education Award.

PREFACE — ARE YOU UNCOMFORTABLE READING X-RAYS?

If you're like me, you received little or no formal training in radiology. Yet, in your day to day work, you may be required to look at x-rays and make decisions based on what you've seen. Like many of our colleagues, you may be frustrated when you see x-rays and aren't sure just what you're looking at. Even if you're not the one ultimately responsible for "reading" an x-ray, you probably want to know more about x-rays than you already do. In other words, my friend, your level of comfort at reading x-rays is less than you'd like it to be!

Fear no more — after reading this book, you **WILL** be comfortable making sense out of most of the common x-rays we use in clinical medicine. X-rays are not as difficult as many people think. It does not require a "PhD" in nuclear physics to make sense out of most films. A few basic principles are *very* important — I'll repeat these often throughout the book. And you **WILL** remember them by the time we're done. If you keep these in mind, and use the approach outlined in this book, the mystery of x-rays will fade.

Have fun,

Mikel

Mikel A. Rothenberg, M.D.
Emergency Care Educator
North Olmsted, Ohio

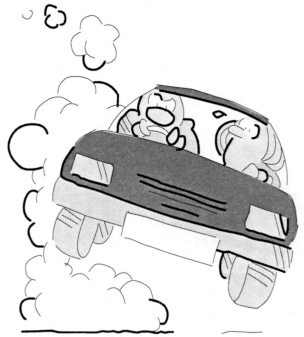

X-rays shouldn't drive you crazy!

Thank you...

I've been working on this book, in one way, shape or form, for the past ten years. I am both incredibly excited, and highly relieved, to have the task completed. It truly represents a dream come true — a "plain English" method of x-ray interpretation for everyone.

I thank my students, who have enthusiastically supported my efforts. Without their encouragement, I might have given up. I especially appreciate the efforts of the following health care professionals who gave me honest and helpful feedback on this final version — Kaye McLain, BSN, MSN; Margie Majure, RN; Linda Brewer, RN, FNP; Paula Clearman, RN, FNP; Alice A. McCann, RN, FNP; Steven F. Williams, BT, ET; Reana M. Uihlein, LPN, CAD.

Dr. Dale Dubin taught me the beauty of simplicity in communication many years ago. His landmark text, "Rapid Interpretation of EKG's," remains the epitome of "user-friendly" learning. If I can communicate my system of x-ray interpretation with anywhere near the success that Dr. Dubin has taught health care providers to make sense out of EKG's, I will have truly accomplished my goal. Thank you, Dale, for your friendship and ongoing support.

Kathleen A. Dubin, JD spent countless hours editing my manuscript. Without her dedication and hard work, this book would have been far less "polished." Thank you, thank you, thank you, Kathleen...

Last, and certainly not least... My family has tolerated my obsessive-compulsive nature above the call of duty. Thank you, Diane, Kara, and Marc. I love and cherish you more than you may ever know.

Mikel A. Rothenberg, M.D.
Emergency Care Educator
North Olmsted, Ohio
March 1, 1998

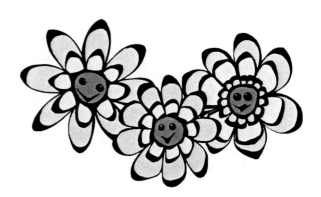

ABOUT PESI

Professional Education Systems, Inc. was founded in 1979. Since that time, more than 800,000 busy professionals have relied on PESI for their continuing education needs, and we have sponsored almost 10,000 seminar days. Longevity and productivity are not the only measures of success, however. We measure our success by the reliability and timeliness of the information we provide you, by the quality of our service to you, and by our number of repeat customers, the cornerstone of our business.

Services provided by PESI include conferences, seminars, workshops, distance education via the telephone and internet, self-study audiocassette/manual packages, in-house training and educational manuals. More information about us can be found at www.pesi.com.

We are sincerely thankful that you have chosen us to fill your information needs. Our mission is to excel at identifying and meeting those needs in the format you desire.

I invite your comments and suggestions to assist us in improving our service to you. Please e-mail me at mhelland@pesi.com or write to me at PESI, Box 1428, Eau Claire, WI 54702.

Sincerely,

Mark Helland

Mark Helland, President
PESI

Visit our web site at www.pesi.com

How To Use
This Book

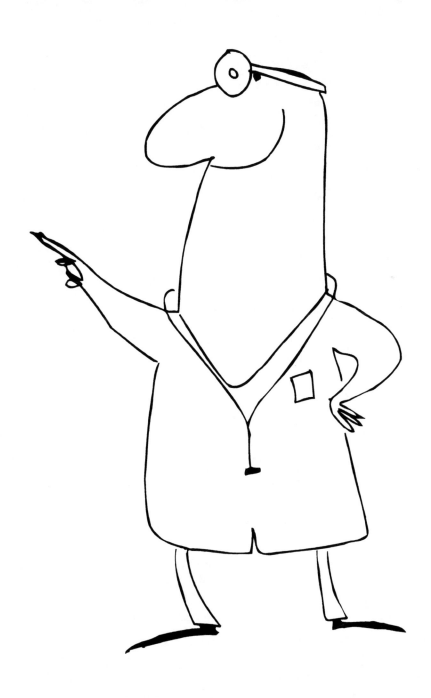

HOW TO USE THIS BOOK

To simplify learning, I've organized this book into six sections:

- **Section 1: Introductory Principles** — This material defines the terms you'll need to know and describes the basics of x-ray interpretation. We discuss a system you can use to understand *any* x-ray. Even if you are already comfortable with x-rays, these principles are the *basis* of this system. If you don't know the system like "the back of your hand," the rest of this book will be "challenging," or worse...

- **Section 2: The Chest and Abdomen** — This section covers the basics of normal chest and abdomen x-rays. You'll learn how to recognize common abnormal conditions, such as lung infiltrates, pleural effusion, and pneumothorax. We'll also discuss tube placement and tumors. No matter what your clinical interest, this section will be helpful to you.

- **Section 3: Mostly Bony Injuries** — Here, we first discuss normal anatomy of the skeletal system. This section then reviews bony and soft tissue injuries to the head, face, neck, pelvis, and extremities. If you work in a setting where you see musculoskeletal trauma, you'll find this information invaluable.

- **Section 4: Let's Review** — At this point, you've covered the "core" material in the book. This section reviews the basic principles you should remember. Here, we use the "programmed learning" approach where you read the question on one half of the page and cover the answer, located on the other side. Little by little, you reinforce what you've learned. This is a good place to go for a general introduction to the "system," and for a periodic refresher.

- **Section 5: More Fun if You're Interested** — These appendices provide didactic material on procedural topics, such as how to order an x-ray, x-ray triage principles, and medicolegal aspects of x-rays. This material is important, but very different from what you actually need to know to interpret an x-ray.

- **Section 6: Additional Reading** — It's impossible to cover everything in an introductory text. I've included a reading list of some reference and more advanced textbooks. Refer to these as you need.

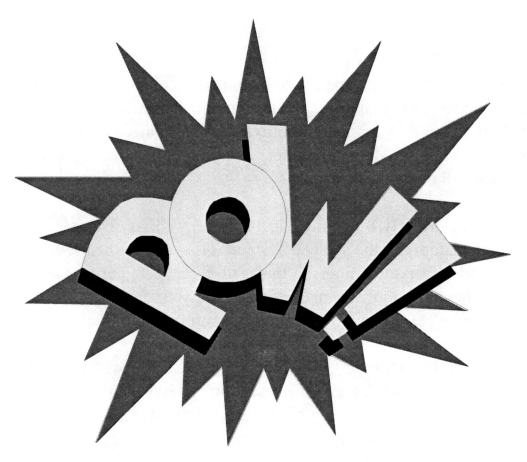

Let's Do It!

UNDERSTANDING X-RAYS:
A PLAIN ENGLISH APPROACH

Table of Contents

By Mikel A. Rothenberg MD

Section 1: Introductory Principles

INTRODUCTION - X-RAYS ARE FUN AND EASY

Chapter Outline...Intro-1
Learning Objectives...Intro-1
The School of Hard Knocks...Intro-2
Plain Films...Intro-3
Plain English..Intro-4
Trust Me - I'm a Doctor...Intro-5
Radiographers Are Your Best Friends...Intro-5
It's All How You View It..Intro-6
X-Rays Are ONE Diagnostic Tool...Intro-7
X-Rays Have Limitations...Intro-8
Friendly Advice..Intro-9

BASIC PRINCIPLES: PHYSICS IS FUN!

Chapter Outline...Basics-1
Learning Objectives...Basics-1
The Basics..Basics-2
X-Ray Talk - Terminology...Basics-2
Rules of the Game..Basics-5
A General Approach to Any X-Ray..Basics-8
Compare to the Normal...Basics-12
Summary - The Basics...Basics-12

Section 2: The Chest and Abdomen

THE CHEST: WE'RE NOT ALL HEART!

Chapter Outline Chest-1
Learning Objectives.. Chest-2
The Normal Chest Film Chest-3
Normal Cardiac Diameter.. Chest-9
An Easy Way to Make Sense of Just About Any Chest Film................. Chest-13
Abnormal Air Shadows Chest-15
    Pneumothorax... Chest-16
    Asthma/COPD Chest-25
Abnormal Water (Fluid) Shadows Chest-26
    Pleural Effusion Chest-27
    Pericardial Effusion Chest-34
    Infiltrates Chest-34
Common Conditions That Cause Infiltrates Chest-42
    Congestive Heart Failure Chest-42
    Noncardiogenic Pulmonary Edema.. Chest-47
    Pneumonia Chest-47
    Pulmonary Embolism Chest-48
    Pulmonary Contusion Chest-48
    Aortic Trauma Chest-49
Abnormal Bones (Trauma).. Chest-50
    Rib Fractures Chest-51
    Sternal and Scapular Fractures Chest-52
    Metastatic Bone Disease Chest-53
Funny Looking Things Chest-53
    Tubes Chest-54
    Lines Chest-56
    Pacers and Leads Chest-58
    Masses Chest-59
    Foreign Bodies Chest-61
Summary - Rules of the Chest... Chest-63

THE ABDOMEN: MOANS AND GROANS

Chapter Outline ABD-1
Learning Objectives ABD-1
The Normal Abdominal Film.. ABD-2
Abnormal Air Shadows.. ABD-4
    Free Intraperitoneal "Air" ABD-5
    Motility Disturbances... ABD-7
Abnormal Water Shadows.. ABD-11
Funny Looking Things... ABD-12

Tubes ABD-12
Foreign Bodies ABD-12
Abnormal Calcifications ABD-13
Summary - Rules of the Abdomen...ABD-17

Section 3: Mostly Bony Injuries

THE BONES: SNAPPY BUT BUT SIMPLE

Outline Bones-1
Learning Objectives...Bones-2
Bony Basics - A Review...Bones-3
Skull and Face Bones-4
The Spine Bones-11
The Upper Extremity Bones-25
The Pelvis and Hips...Bones-45
The Lower Extremity Bones-50
Summary - Bone Rules...Bones-60

Section 4: Let's Review

IMPORTANT! Instructions ....Let's Review-1
The Basics ....Let's Review-2
X-Rays...Let's Review-3
The Chest..Let's Review-12
The Abdomen ....Let's Review-53
Bones ....Let's Review-66
Unknowns..Let's Review-99

Section 5: More Fun If You're Interested

Requisitions: How to Order X-Rays Without Getting a Migraine . . . .More Fun-1
Patient Preparation and Care - My Patients Don't "Code" in X-Ray!................More Fun-2
Radiographic Decision-Making - Is There a Method to Our Madness?............More Fun-4
X-Ray Triage - A Great Timesaver . . . .More Fun-6
Medical-Legal Aspects of X-Rays - How to Avoid the Thrill of a Summons
and The Agony of a Deposition! ....More Fun-7

Section 6: Additional Reading

Additional Reading Page-1
Index to Chapters...Index-1
Thank You Index-6

Section 1:

Introductory Principles

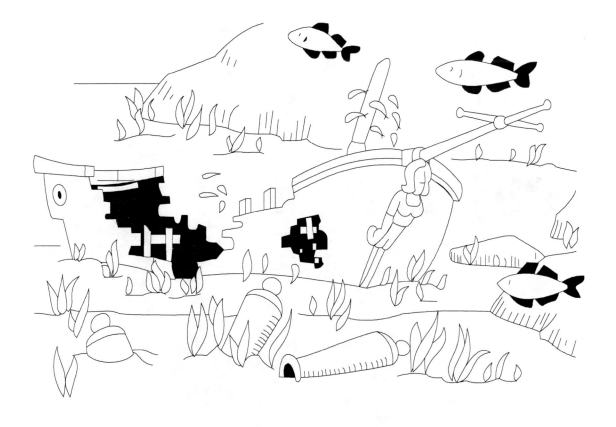

Introduction:

X-Rays Are Fun and Easy!

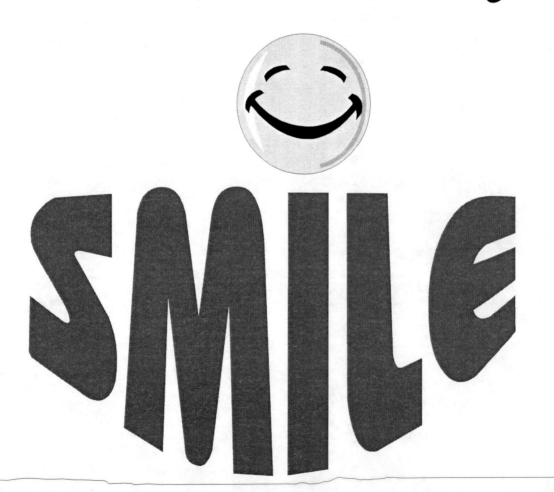

INTRODUCTION — X-RAYS ARE FUN AND EASY!

CHAPTER OUTLINE

Introduction — X-Rays are Fun and Easy!
  The School of Hard Knocks
  Plain Films
  Plain English
  Trust Me — I'm a Doctor
  Radiographers Are Your Best Friends
  It's All How You View It
  X-Rays Are <u>One</u> Diagnostic Tool
  X-Rays Have Limitations
  Friendly Advice

LEARNING OBJECTIVES

After completing this chapter, you'll be able to:

1. Appreciate the need for a reliable, but simple, system for making sense out of just about any x-ray.

2. Define the term "plain x-rays."

3. Explain the need to ask the radiographer (x-ray technologist) for help.

4. Describe the basic principles regarding patient positioning and different x-ray views.

5. Explain why making a diagnosis from an x-ray alone is often difficult.

THE SCHOOL OF HARD KNOCKS

If you're like me, you didn't get much formal education in how to make sense out of x-rays during your professional training. In fact, most of what I know after twenty years of medical practice is thanks to advice from friends, independent reading, and mostly, the "school of hard knocks." Several years ago, it hit me — x-rays just aren't as confusing as I had been led to believe. I worked out a system, in "plain English," to make sense out of just about any plain x-ray film that I came across. I tried my little acronyms and "silly sayings" out on friends and colleagues — and they liked it!

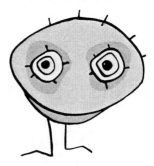

Keep it simple, silly!

After teaching thousands of health care professionals the same system for the past ten years, I decided to put it in writing. My hope is that even more people will come to realize how fun looking at x-rays can be — and how easy it really is, if you just have a system! I think that the most powerful testament to the fact that this system *really* works is the people who come up to me years later and thank me. Despite all their advanced education, they still found that simple words, like "Bones are smooth, when they're not smooth they're broken," work best!

Fear no more — after reading this book, you **WILL** be comfortable making sense out of most of the common x-rays we use in clinical medicine. As clinicians, we want to integrate the x-ray findings into our "data base" when

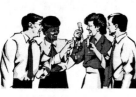

For Adults

Only!

we care for patients. Therefore, this book is clinically-oriented. You will be able to take the techniques taught here and use them directly in your day-to-day practice. Though many of the principles I teach here are useful in pediatric films, I've limited the discussion to adults. Pediatric radiology is a complete subspeciality in and of itself.

X-rays are not as difficult as many people think. It does not require a "PhD" in nuclear physics to make sense out of most films. There are a few basic principles that are very important — I'll repeat these many times throughout the book. And you *WILL* remember them by the time we're done. If you keep these in mind, and use the approach outlined in this book, the mystery of x-rays will fade.

The *entire* system consists of two definitions, three rules, and one acronym. These will become perfectly clear as you read on. Whenever the going gets rough, remember that virtually *any* x-ray looks the way it does because of these principles. Don't make something difficult that really isn't...

REMEMBER — the entire system depends upon only two definitions, three rules, and one acronym!

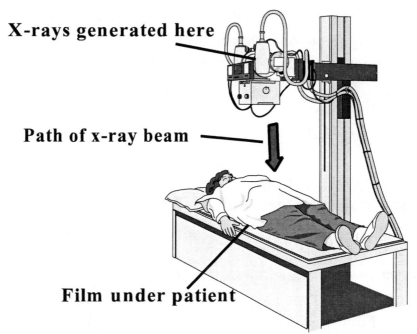

X-rays generated here

Path of x-ray beam

Film under patient

The way to get really good at making sense out of x-rays is: Look at a lot of x-rays! Keep practicing — constantly challenge yourself to improve your skills and comfort level. Before you know it, you'll find yourself seeing things on x-rays that you never did before.

PLAIN FILMS

We're only going to talk about "plain" x-ray films. Since I promised that everything I write here will be one hundred percent perfectly clear, let's define "plain film." By this, I mean the film generated when the patient stands (or sits or lies) in the path of the x-ray beam, with a film plate on the other side. The x-rays pass through the patient, to at least some extent (which we'll talk more about later on), and hit the film. The film is developed in a processor and, *voilá*, we have a plain x-ray. This is the easiest of any of the currently available radiological processes.

Sure, CT scans, ultrasound, MRI, nuclear scans, and SPECT scans are very important — but first things first. Once you feel very comfortable with plain XR's, the other imaging modalities are far easier to understand. Every now and then, I'll throw in a little bit of information incorporating use of one of these "fancier" tests so you can see how the newer tests and the "good old" plain x-rays complement each other.

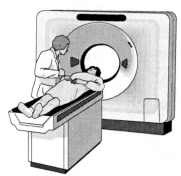

PLAIN ENGLISH

I tend to talk "plain English" to just about everyone, regardless of their title or the initials after their name. And, that's the way I write as well... just as if we were sitting down and talking it over. Or, like you were in one of my many classes. Most people appreciate a straightforward and easy-to-understand approach. Trust me (I'm a doctor, after all!) — I don't ever mean to be condescending or "talk down" to anyone — I've just found that the simple approach is best. *PLEASE* — give it a try, even if you're a little unsure at first. If you follow my system, I can almost guarantee that you'll be able to make sense out of nearly 95% of common plain x-rays that you will ever see — no matter who you are, where you practice, or the initials after your name...

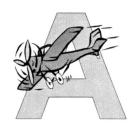

"Plain English"

TRUST ME — I'M A DOCTOR

I urge you temporarily to forget *everything* you ever knew about x-rays and re-learn it my way. The reason? Because I know it will work for you. I use a lot of silly terms to make things easy to remember as well as fun. Again, please don't take this the wrong way — my experience of over twenty years has proven that having fun and using crazy mnemonics work better than dry, overly-didactic information. Let's face it — x-rays can be incredibly boring! *We* are going to have fun!

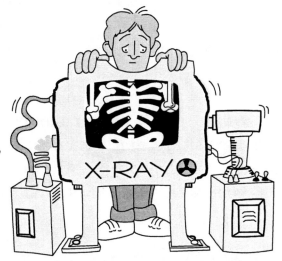

X-rays are fun and easy!!

RADIOGRAPHERS ARE YOUR BEST FRIENDS

By the way — my formal training was in internal medicine and critical care — I'm *not* a radiologist or a radiographer (radiologic technologist). Most of the time, I don't have the *slightest idea* as to the technical aspects of taking x-rays. Readers who are experts in this area, welcome! I feel strongly about deferring to you. I will be able to give you lots of little hints to improve your interpretative skills, but I always confer with the "tech" on which films to do — and I feel that all of us non-tech types should do the same! By the way — there has been a lot of recent controversy over the proper terminology for the radiologic

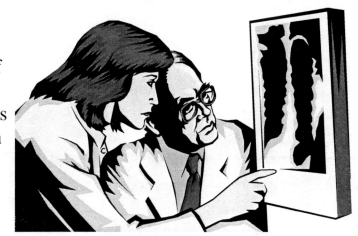

Work together as a team...

technologist. With sincere respect, I use the terms "x-ray tech," "radiology tech," "radiologic technologist," and "radiographer" interchangeably. In my mind, they *all* refer to the same highly-skilled professional who has dug me out of trouble many times!

This book is *not* designed to make you a "one-day radiologist." I regularly utilize the expertise of the radiologist. At the same time, *numerous* health care providers *regularly* interpret x-rays *without* the contemporaneous assistance of a radiologist, who only provides the "official reading" later. This book is for you. I invite your comments and input.

IT'S ALL HOW YOU VIEW IT

> **One view is always one view too few!**

Most of us know what "posterior-anterior" and "lateral" mean. But there are so many views, and so many names, it's just not worth memorizing them unless this knowledge is part of what you do every day — ask the radiographer for help! The only tips I can offer on "technical aspects" are these:

Pull out the "bellows" in your mind to imagine the film in three dimensions...

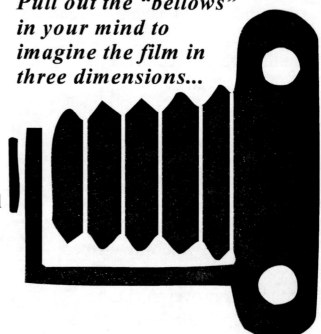

- "One view is always one view too few!" — get at least two views at right angles to each other — by doing this, you can put things into three-dimensional perspective. Remember, x-rays are a one-dimensional representation of a three-dimensional patient. Mentally, we need to reverse this fact —

sort of like an old bellows camera... you should "pull out" the structures in your mind and place them into a three-dimensional perspective.

- By moving a patient, you can sometimes see abnormalities that would otherwise remain subtle or not visible. A good example of this is a hairline fracture of the fibula. It is often missed in the standard "tib-fib" film, but may be easily seen by rotating the leg ever so slightly. Many of these "variant" views are not formally named. Most radiographers are skilled at obtaining them anyway.

- Make sure you see what you need to get the information you're looking for. For example, if the patient hurts over the seventh cervical vertebra (C7) and the lateral neck x-ray only shows C1 - C5, *somebody's* got a problem!

- ASK, ASK, ASK for suggestions on alternative positions and imaging modalities to maximize the information you get from x-rays.

X-RAYS ARE <u>ONE</u> DIAGNOSTIC TOOL

A final, but very important word — XR's are a *diagnostic tool*. The last thing I want you to come away with is the idea that you can look at any x-ray and *immediately* make a *diagnosis*. X-rays are just one of many pieces of information that clinicians utilize to reach conclusions — others include lab, history, physical, other studies, and one's own "gut feelings." True, if a patient hurts an ankle and the XR shows the bones in twenty pieces, you can pretty safely call "ankle fracture." On the other hand, lots of things cause funny-looking shadows on the chest x-ray. If you simply memorize the typical pattern of a community-acquired pneumococcal pneumonia, for example, you're going to be fooled (and the patient might be compromised) if something else is going on that looks the same on the film. In fact, I can come up with at least two other conditions that *may* cause an identical x-ray appearance to several of the "classic pictures" that I have read about and heard of over the years!

Rather than jumping to a diagnosis, please try it my way. Look at the film, describe what you see, understand what causes it to look the way it does, *then* consider what the causes may be. Finally, use all the clinical information available to you to formulate a differential diagnosis (list of diagnostic possibilities).

X-RAYS HAVE LIMITATIONS

Done properly, x-rays reveal much important information. Like any test, they also have their limitations. Many of us were taught that x-rays "make or break" a diagnosis, especially when we look at bone films (pardon the pun!). This is not always the case:

- Sometimes abnormalities don't initially show on the x-ray.

- Sometimes *we* miss an abnormality on the x-ray.

- Sometimes *the radiologist* misses an abnormality on the x-ray.

- A normal x-ray does not always mean a "normal" patient.

Don't jump to conclusions...

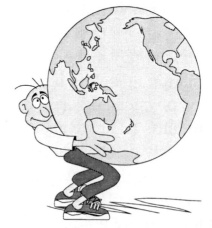

There are many cases where the patient is quite ill and the x-rays are "normal." Use the x-ray as an adjunct to your clinical judgement. Patients with *pneumocystis carinii* pneumonia, for example, often present with a normal or nondescript chest x-ray. The clue is a sick, hypoxic patient with a relatively benign-appearing chest film.

Similarly, patients with fractures of the navicular bone of the wrist commonly have normal plain films. Sometimes, even *special* navicular films appear normal. Treat the patient based on your clinical impression. Missed navicular fractures have serious consequences — untreated, the distal fragment may develop avascular necrosis. The patient then suffers chronic osteoarthritis of the hand.

FRIENDLY ADVICE

When we begin to analyze x-rays systematically, our first tendency is to over-read them. In other words, everything looks abnormal! This is common — with time, you'll learn to recognize how overlapping shadows can sometimes mimic abnormalities. When in doubt, ask. Don't despair if you question something on a film that turns out to be normal. Be pleased that you were observant enough to see a questionable shadow in the first place!

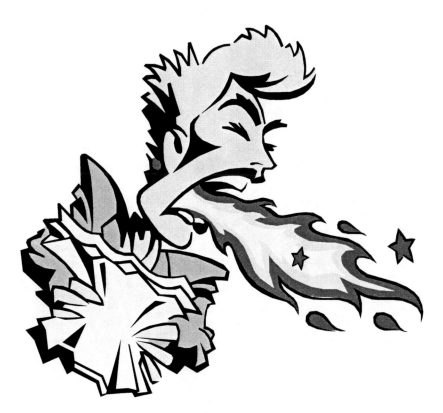

"Friendly" advice...

Basic Principles:

Physics Is Fun!

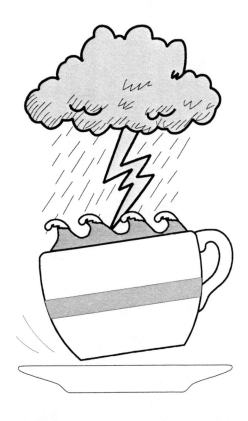

BASIC PRINCIPLES — PHYSICS IS FUN!

CHAPTER OUTLINE

Basic Principles — Physics is Fun!
    The Basics
    X-Ray Talk — Terminology
    Rules of the Game
    A General Approach to Any X-Ray
    Compare to the Normal
    Summary — The Basics

LEARNING OBJECTIVES

After completing this chapter, you'll be able to:

1.   Define the term roentgen.

2.   Define the terms radiopaque and radiolucent.

3.   Describe the expected appearance of radiopaque and radiolucent materials on a plain x-ray.

4.   Understand and explain why various materials appear as they do on a plain x-ray.

5.   Understand and explain the reasons for the appearance of interfaces.

6.   Formulate and describe a general approach to make sense out of nearly any x-ray.

7.   Understand and explain the importance of comparing an unknown x-ray to a known normal film.

THE BASICS

As we were growing up, most of us learned at one time or the other that x-rays don't go through lead. If you understand this principle, then you know at least half of the physics necessary to make sense out of x-ray films! X-rays are a form of electromagnetic energy and penetrate materials to a variable degree, depending upon their "radiographic density." Please remember that "radiographic density" does *not* necessarily correlate with "density" as we think of it — more on this in a bit. The international unit of x-ray energy is the **roentgen**, abbreviated "R." Just to show how rough all of this is, guess who it was named after. You're right — Dr. (Conrad) Roentgen!

X-RAY TALK — TERMINOLOGY

The most powerful technique to understand x-rays is to be able to figure out *why* any given film looks as it does. With practice and a little background, this task becomes relatively simple. First of all, though, you *must* know the proper terminology. Without the right "talk," you won't be able to "walk the right walk"!

The two most important words in "x-ray talk" are **radiopaque**, also known as "radiodense," and **radiolucent**. *Radiopaque materials* resist the passage of x-rays through them. Imagine an x-ray beam aimed at a cube of lead — a very radiopaque object. If we place a film plate on the other side and turn on the beam, very few x-rays will get

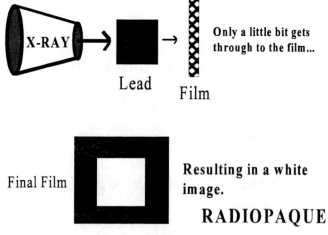

through the lead. For right now, assume that there will be at least a little scatter of the radiation and some *will* get though, but not very many. So, very few x-rays will hit the film — agreed? Now, "shadows" of radiopaque materials appear *white* on plain x-rays. In other words, areas of the film that don't get hit by a lot of x-rays are white. So, the whiter the shadow, the more *radiopaque* or *radiodense* is the material it represents.

Think about it — many of you have already looked at x-ray films and *know* that shadows of bones are whitish. Makes sense, doesn't it, since bones are radiopaque. Also consider barium contrast studies — the contrast material is highly radiopaque, causing a white shadow on the final film. Again, remember we're referring to the *radiological density*, not the actual mass density of a material. For example, liquid contrast material is very dense from a radiographic point of view (and appears what "color" on the plain film?)... yet, it is a liquid. Solid materials such as clay are far more dense than liquid contrast material, but appear relatively radiolucent when x-rayed.

Radiolucent materials have the opposite property — they allow the passage of x-rays to a variable degree, depending on their radiodensity. Probably the most radiolucent material around us is air. If we imagine aiming our x-ray beam through air towards a film plate, what happens? This time, many of the x-rays get through air — because it's so radiolucent. So, lots of x-rays hit the film and form a *dark* shadow. The more x-rays that hit the film, the darker the shadow. So, we can conclude that *dark shadows* represent materials that are very radiolucent.

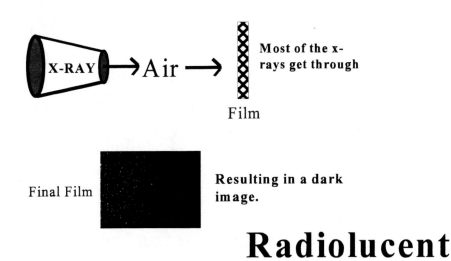

Radiolucent

Medically speaking, things in the body aren't just black and white. There is a spectrum of radiographic densities ranging from highly radiopaque (bones) to very radiolucent (gas and fat). For most of the intermediate density tissues, we're actually talking about different "shades of grey" rather than simply "real black" or "real white." I find it far easier to take artistic liberty and use the word "colors" to refer to the

REMEMBER — **Radiopaque materials resist the passage of x-rays, resulting in white shadows. Radiolucent materials allow x-rays to pass, leading to dark (black) shadows. The *more* x-rays that hit a film, the darker the shadow; the *fewer* that hit it, the lighter the shadow. These are the *two* definitions you must know!**

various shades of black, grey, and white seen in an x-ray. It just fits in better with an easy-going "plain English" conversation. So, when I talk about different "colors" on the x-ray, I really mean different shades of grey, white, or black.

Imagine a cross-section of a limb — for now, we'll make it very simple and look at three areas as seen by an x-ray. First of all, the bones. These offer a fair amount of resistance to the passage of x-rays, allowing only a few to hit the film below. The shadow of the bones is then, what color? Of course, it's

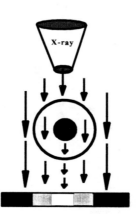

Radiolucent (air around arm)

Intermediate ("guts" of arm)

Radiopaque (bones)

white because bones are radiopaque — shadows of radiopaque structures appear white on the final film because very few x-rays get through the radiodense bone to hit the film plate. On the other hand, look at the rim of air surrounding the limb. Gas is radiolucent — by allowing lots of x-rays through to hit the film plate, the shadow of the air is dark. Remember, the more x-rays that hit the film plate, the darker the shadow. Finally, consider the "guts" of the limb. These include the muscles, tendons, fascia, blood vessels, nerves, and other structures that aren't part of the bones. Taken together, they are more radiopaque than air but less than bone — do you agree? Then they should appear as an intermediate density or "color" on the x-ray, which they do. Make sure you clearly understand *why* the cross-sectional view of our simplified limb looks as it does on x-ray before you move on...

RULES OF THE GAME

The power and beauty of this system is that you can apply it to any x-ray in just about any professional setting. All you need to remember are three basic rules. Simple as they are, be sure that you're comfortable with these rules. They truly form the basis

REMEMBER — **The "colors" of an x-ray reflect a spectrum of shadows ranging from very dark (highly radiolucent) to very light (highly radiopaque), and everything between (different shades of grey).**

from which all understanding of x-rays comes. Practice until you can summarize them in your sleep! Here are the rules:

- At the point where two materials of different radiographic densities meet, there is a **border**. Others prefer the terms "interface" or "line," and that's fine. Just understand that when you see a border, interface, or line on an x-ray, it represents the meeting point of two

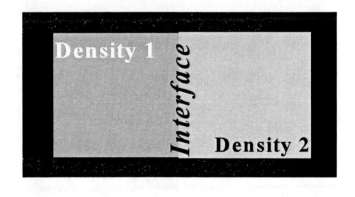

radiographically different materials. The easy way to remember this is the name "Bill": "B" stands for border, "I" for interface, and the "L," for line. On a plain x-ray, different-colored shadows represent materials of different radiographic densities — period! And, at the point where they meet, you see "BILL"!

- The degree of clarity or sharpness of "BILL" depends on the difference in densities between the two materials. If they differ widely (e.g., air and lead), "BILL" is quite *sharp* or clear. The more alike the densities, the *foggier* or less clear "BILL" becomes.

> *REMEMBER* — On the x-ray, a border, interface, or line indicates the meeting point of materials of different radiographic density. We fondly refer to this concept as "BILL"! If the densities differ widely, "BILL" is sharp; the more alike the densities, the fuzzier is "BILL."

- At the point where two materials of the *same* radiographic density meet there is no "BILL"! Stated somewhat differently, if two materials of the same radiographic density meet, any pre-existing border, interface, or line disappears. Imagine the border of the heart on a chest x-ray.

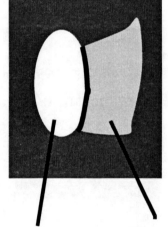

Normally, there is an interface between the heart and the lungs...

Heart   Lungs

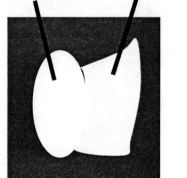

The border disappears where the lung fills with fluid...

If the lungs fill with fluid, which has the same density as that of the heart, "BILL" disappears (assuming enough fluid is present). We'll use this principle over and over again to help determine the presence of abnormal collections of fluid in various areas of the body (e.g., lung infiltrates, pleural effusions, ascites, abdominal abscesses).

Now, let's put these rules to the test. Look at the "x-ray" figure below and tell me what you see:

I bet you said "a square," didn't you? Most people do — and you've just given me a *diagnosis*, not a *description* of what you saw. This is precisely what makes x-rays so difficult for people — they try to memorize the x-ray appearance of all sorts of things, including a white square! I *insist* (please!!) that you try it my way — describe *what you see*, then understand *why it looks the way it does*, and only then venture a guess as to what it could be (diagnosis). I know that this may sound silly at first, but if you have the *method* down, when the film isn't so obvious, you can approach it systematically and things make sense.

Using the system, the proper way to describe the object in the figure might be as follows:

> A "white square" — meaning that not many x-rays have hit the film. So, the object the square represents is what? Fairly radiopaque — it

doesn't let many x-rays through. I also know it's radiopaque because it is very "white," and forms a sharp border with the surrounding air (dark area).

There is *no way* that you can determine whether the object is metal, radiopaque contrast liquid in a plastic mold, or a contrast-impregnated implant — at least by just looking at the x-ray. So, resist your temptation to tell me we're looking at a metal square. Maybe not — the only "sure" bet is that we're looking at a radiopaque object in the shape of a square. Now, let's try one more time — look at the next x-ray figure and tell me what you see.

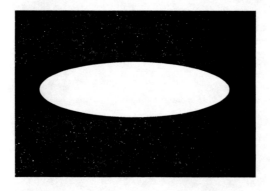

Great! It's an oval-shaped white shadow. Not many x-rays have hit the film, resulting in a white color, indicating that the shadow represents a radiopaque object. Could be just about anything, as long as it's radiopaque.

A GENERAL APPROACH TO ANY X-RAY

Please be absolutely certain you understand the principles above before reading this section. Once you do, you can apply them to just about any film anywhere. When you look at an x-ray, I suggest a two-prong approach similar to the way we approach patients clinically. In the emergency department, for example, my first responsibility is to make sure the patient doesn't have a life-threatening problem I've gotta fix immediately! This is called the **primary survey**. Once things are stabilized, I proceed to a more detailed evaluation, the **secondary survey**.

Applying this approach to the x-ray, you should first do a "**quick scan**" looking for what I fondly refer to as "Rothenberg Readable X-Rays." I say that with a big smile on my face and am referring to obvious abnormalities or deviations. You might want to call these "aha phenomena," as they tend to evoke the words "aha!" from us. Another way to think of this is: "Do I like what I see? Would I want to be the 'proud owner' of this film?"

There is even an acronym to remember what to look for, **"BSO"**:

> **B** — **bony** abnormalities; for example, is the clavicle in several pieces?

> **S** — **soft tissue** abnormalities; for example, is one side of the chest white and the other dark? Is the heart on the correct side of the thorax?

> **O** — **other obvious** problems; for example, is there a huge radiopaque foreign body in the abdomen?

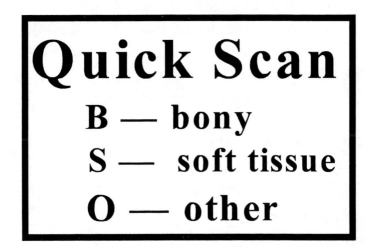

Once you've finished the "quick scan," the next step is to study the film in detail. It's important that you carefully evaluate several aspects of *any film* you look at. To remember what's really important, try the following acronym: **I Quit And Wanna Be Free!!** Say this to yourself ten times now! Repeat it again five times in the morning, at noon, and at night for two weeks. After that, you'll never again forget *anything* that's important in making sense out of any x-ray. More specifically...

I — *Identify* the film; at best, it's "poor form" to make a clinical decision based on the wrong patient's x-ray! Though it sounds real silly, such an error occurs more commonly than any of us would care to admit.

Q — *Quality* of the film; radiographers take pride in producing the very best films possible under the circumstances. It's important for all of us to work together to be certain that the film allows us to obtain as much information as possible. For example, a lateral film of the cervical spine *must* include all seven cervical vertebrae and preferably T1 as well. Otherwise, the likelihood of missing a subtle fracture or malalignment increases greatly.

A — *Air* (gas) shadows; gases are radiolucent and appear dark on x-rays. The only thing that looks similar, at least from a medical point of view, is fat. When you see a dark shadow, it's usually either gas or fat. "Air" shadows are most important when we are looking at the lungs and abdomen, but abnormal collections of gas may occur anywhere in the body (e.g., gas gangrene in the foot).

W — *Water* shadows; fluid (liquid) is relatively radiopaque and appears whitish on the x-ray. Depending on the film, "water shadows" may be very important (heart and lungs) or of little significance (fractured ankle).

B — *Bone* shadows; sometimes, the intent of the film is to look at the bones specifically (e.g., shoulder or AC joint). Other times, the bones are well seen even when evaluating them is not your primary intent (e.g., chest and abdomen x-rays). This portion of the acronym reminds you not to forget about the bones. A common example of this principle is our tendency to "zero in" on the lungs when looking at a chest x-ray. By remembering "I Quit And Wanna *Be* Free," you remember to look at the clavicles, ribs, and scapulae as well. I know of at least four previously unsuspected scapular fractures that were only picked up using this method. Everyone else was busy looking at the lungs for a pneumothorax that wasn't there.

F —   *Funny-looking things*; various shadows that are part of our normal anatomy (e.g., nipple shadows) can create much confusion. A typical (and serious) error that sometimes occurs is when a unilateral round shadow on a chest x-ray is assumed to be from the nipple and later turns out to be lung cancer. This part of the acronym also covers calcifications of all kinds — malignant, degenerative, and infectious — as well as x-rays done for endotracheal tube or central line placement.

I Quit And Wanna Be Free!

Identify
Quality
Air shadows
Water shadows
Bone shadows
Funny-looking things

COMPARE TO THE NORMAL

One of the most helpful techniques in making sense out of x-rays is to compare the patient's film to a known normal. In many films, you can actually use the same film as a comparison view. For example, a routine pelvis film should show both hips, making comparison to find subtle hip fractures much easier. As we'll see, the chest x-ray offers numerous opportunities to take advantage of the body's symmetry, as does the pelvis film. And, use of comparison films in pediatric bony trauma is *very* common.

The System

- **2 definitions (radiopaque, radiolucent)**

- **3 rules ("BILL")**

- **1 acronym ("I Quit And Wanna Be Free!")**

SUMMARY — THE BASICS

Now, I've given you all the foundation material you'll ever need to make sense out of nearly any x-ray. Keep these principles in mind:

- Radiopaque materials prevent the passage of x-rays, leading to white shadows.

- Radiolucent materials allow the passage of x-rays, leading to dark shadows.

- Most materials fall somewhere in between "white and black," reflecting some degree of either radiopacity or radiolucency, leading to "grey" shadows.

- The more x-rays that hit a film, the darker the shadow; the fewer, the lighter the shadow.

- A border, interface, or line ("BILL") indicates the meeting point of materials of different radiographical densities. Wide differences in density lead to sharp borders while similar densities result in fuzzier borders.

- At the point where materials of the *same* radiographic density meet, there is no border.

- When looking at an x-ray, first do a "quick scan" (BSO).

- Then, do a more detailed analysis remembering **"I Quit And Wanna Be Free!"**

- Remember to compare the unknown film to a known normal; sometimes, you can use the same film for comparison (e.g., bilateral hips on a pelvis film).

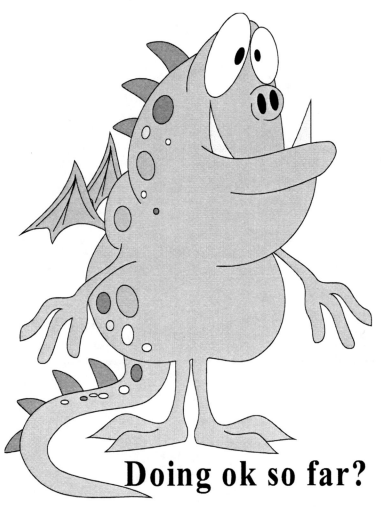

Doing ok so far?

Section 2:

The Chest and Abdomen

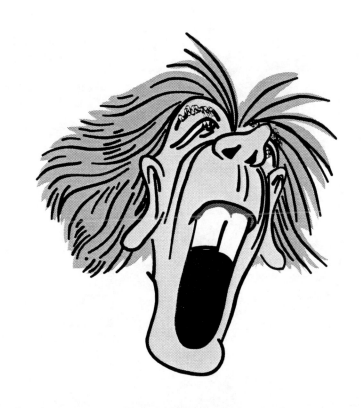

The Chest:

We're Not All Heart!

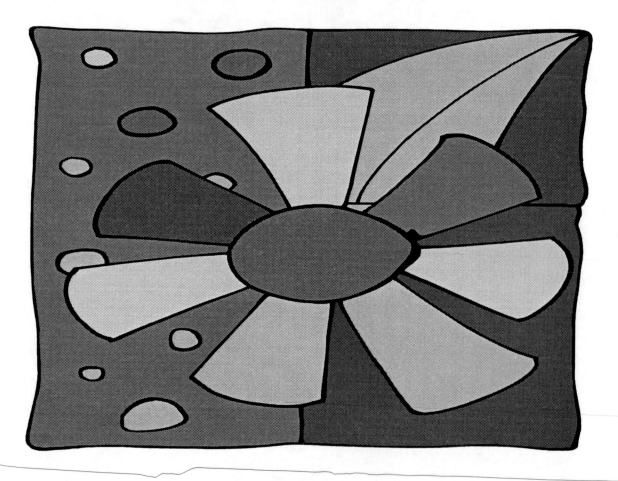

THE CHEST — WE'RE NOT ALL HEART!

CHAPTER OUTLINE

The Chest — We're Not All Heart!
    The Normal Chest Film
        The Chest Tree
        The Diaphragm Shadows
        The Costophrenic Angles
        The Heart
        The Hilar Markings
        The Lung Markings
    An Easy Way to Make Sense of Just About Any Chest Film
    Abnormal Air (Gas) Shadows
        Pneumothorax
        Ruptured Diaphragm
        Asthma/COPD
    Abnormal Water (Fluid) Shadows
        Pleural Effusion
        Pericardial Effusion
        Infiltrates
        Common Conditions that Cause Infiltrates
            Congestive Heart Failure
            Noncardiogenic Pulmonary Edema
            Pneumonia
            Pulmonary Embolism
            Pulmonary Contusion
            Aortic Trauma
    Abnormal Bones (Trauma)
        Rib Fractures
        Sternal and Scapular Fractures
        Metastatic Disease
    Funny Looking Things
        Tubes

Lines
Pacers and Leads
Masses
Foreign Bodies
Summary — Rules of the Chest

LEARNING OBJECTIVES

After completing this chapter, you'll be able to:

1. Describe the appearance of a normal chest x-ray.

2. Describe and recognize abnormal collections of air (gas) seen on the chest x-ray.

3. Describe and recognize abnormal collections of fluid seen on the chest x-ray.

4. Identify common chest x-ray features of the following conditions: congestive heart failure, pulmonary edema, pneumonia, aortic aneurysm, asthma, COPD.

5. Analyze a chest x-ray and judge if the following devices are in their proper position: CVP/central venous line, ET tube, Swan-Ganz catheter, intra-cardiac pacemakers, chest tube.

6. Recognize and describe the role of the chest x-ray in diagnosis of the following traumatic conditions: rib fracture, sternum fracture, pulmonary contusion, aortic tear, rupture of the diaphragm.

THE NORMAL CHEST FILM

First, I'm going to go over selected parts of the normal chest film in detail. Afterwards, I will present three rules that cover just about everything you will *ever* need to make sense out of most chest x-rays. As throughout this book, we will look at only those selected views that are likely to be of the most diagnostic value.

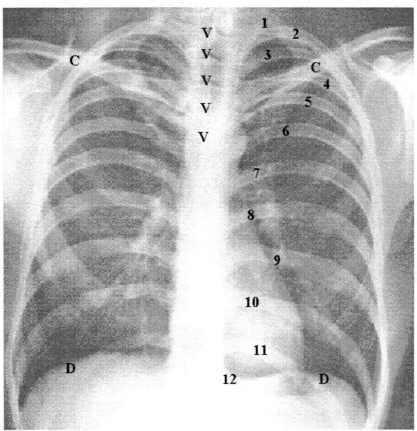

Figure C-1 — Normal Chest Film

The chest tree — Somewhat metaphorically speaking, I find it very helpful to think initially of the normal chest x-ray as a tree. The trunk of the tree is the vertebral column. Vertebral interspaces (labeled "V" in the diagram) should be just barely visible at least to the level of the clavicle. Depending upon the exposure of the film, they may be visible along the entire thoracic spine. You *should not* be able to see well-defined vertebral bodies — if you do, the film is overexposed (overpenetrated). The base of the tree consists of the diaphragm shadows (labeled "D" in the diagram) — more on these shortly.

The branches of the tree are the clavicles (labeled "C" in the diagram) and the twelve ribs. Counting ribs is always a challenging adventure the first few times around. Look at the skeleton in Figure C-1. Remember that in three dimensions, the first and second ribs are superior to the clavicle. Make a habit out of practicing on every chest film you look at. I've numbered the ribs on the normal PA film for your reference.

Using the "chest tree" model, it's relatively easy to determine the *quality* of a standard AP or PA chest film. Recently, I learned a neat acronym: "RIP" (rest in peace) or rotation, inspiration, and penetration:

- Rotation — the orientation of the clavicles should be equal on both sides of the vertebrae, nearly forming a cross. Otherwise, the x-ray beam is not passing perpendicular to the AP plane of the patient.

- Inspiration — the routine chest film is taken during full inspiration. If the patient does not take in an adequate breath, the lungs are not expanded to the normal extent. The result? The lung tissue is denser, fewer x-rays get through, so fewer hit the film, and the shadows are *whiter* than they should be. This artificial increase in density misleads us into thinking there are shadows in the lung fields (e.g., infiltrates — see below) that would *not* be present in a properly-taken film. In addition, the diaphragm does not move inferiorly as far as it normally should, causing a falsely-enlarged cardiac silhouette (see below). The easiest way to decide if a patient's inspiration was adequate or not is to count the ribs. In a good film, you should be able

> **REMEMBER — If you don't see at least eight ribs, it's a poor inspiratory effort.**

to count *at least* eight ribs; most radiographers strive for at least ten, though. If you don't see at least eight ribs, it's a poor inspiratory effort.

- Penetration — a fancy x-ray term for "exposure." An over-penetrated (overexposed) film means that the setting on the x-ray machine was too *high* resulting in *too many* beams passing through the patient and hitting the film. The effect, of course, is *too dark* a shadow. Under-penetration (underexposed) is the opposite — the "juice" is turned down too low and *not enough* x-rays get through to cause a proper image. This leads to *fewer* than expected x-rays hitting the film, and thus, in a *whiter* shadow than normal. Over-penetration of a chest film causes the lung fields to look darker than normal and may obliterate a subtle opacity. Under-penetration, on the other hand, makes the lung fields *lighter* than normal and may lead to the false appearance of lung masses or infiltrates.

The easiest way to tell if a chest film is properly penetrated is to look at the trunk of the tree — the vertebral column. Normally, below the clavicles you should *just* be able to make out the interspaces and see little, if any, of the vertebral body outline. If the lateral margins of the vertebral bodies are well-defined, as in a properly exposed AP thoracic spine film, the x-ray is over-penetrated!

> ## Chest X-Ray Technique
>
> **R** — Rotation (clavicles and vertebrae form a cross)
>
> **I** — Inspiration (minimum of 8 ribs visible)
>
> **P** — Penetration (interspaces visible; thoracic vertebral bodies *not* well-defined)

The diaphragm shadows — At the base of the tree lie the diaphragm shadows. Note, I did not say "the diaphragm." Am I being picky? I think not. Anatomically speaking, the diaphragm is pretty darn thin. Yet, the shadow on the chest film we sometimes call "the diaphragm" is often a couple inches thick. Obviously, we're not looking at just the diaphragm.

Think about it — if you're an x-ray beam going through that part of the body, through which structures will you pass? The skin, muscles, ribs, diaphragm, liver, and retroperitoneal structures. Normally, the liver and the right diaphragm (more properly called **hemidiaphragm**) are right up next to each other. Since both have the same radiographic density, would you expect to see an interface? No! So the "diaphragm shadow" on the right is actually a

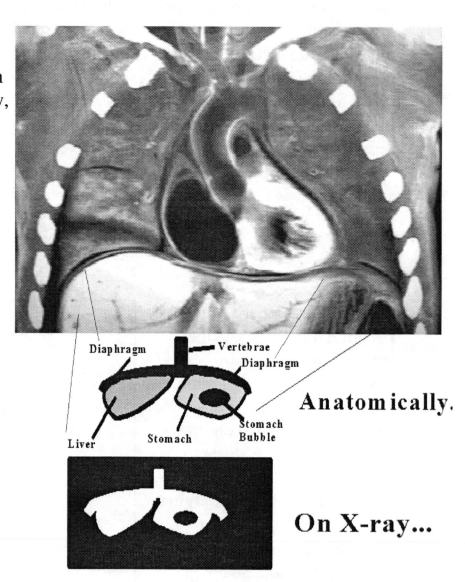

Figure C-2 — Why the diaphragm should never be "paper-thin"

combination of the diaphragm and liver (maybe we should change the name to the "liver shadow"???). Similarly, the "diaphragm shadow" on the patient's left is a combination of left hemidiaphragm, spleen, and stomach.

Often, you can see the gas bubble in the stomach as well. Knowing that gas is radiolucent, what "color" would you expect the "stomach bubble" to appear?

The right hemidiaphragm is normally a bit higher (one to two cm) than the left, due to the size of the liver. If the left side appears higher, or the right side is more than one or two cm higher than the left, the film is abnormal. Possible explanations are many — ruptured diaphragm, phrenic nerve paralysis, organomegaly, congenital abnormality. Often, it is difficult to determine the reasons from the x-ray alone.

> **_REMEMBER_ — If the diaphragm is paper-thin, then there's gotta be free air within... the peritoneal cavity!**

The diaphragm should never be paper-thin. If the diaphragm shadow on either or both sides appears paper-thin, the film is abnormal. Most likely, a "paper-thin diaphragm" indicates free intraperitoneal "air," i.e., gas from a ruptured hollow viscus. More about this in "The Abdomen..."

The costophrenic angles — Bilaterally, the diaphragm shadow meets an imaginary vertical line through the rib shadows along the edge of each hemithorax. Together, the shadow and this "line" define the costophrenic angle. On the PA or AP film, _the costophrenic angles should always be sharp._ Blunting (clouding) of either

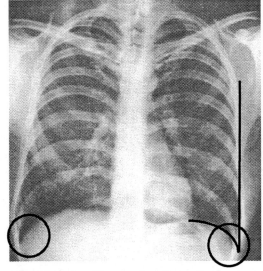

Costophrenic Angles
Figure C-3

> **_REMEMBER_ — The costophrenic angles should be sharp. If they're not, suspect a pleural effusion. Don't be misled by overlapping _normal_ rib shadows!**

angle is an early sign of fluid in the pleural cavity (pleural effusion). Remember, you are still usually able to see overlapping shadows of the ribs in the area of the costophrenic angles — this is *normal*.

The heart — Many books point out in detail the external structures of the heart. It's difficult to try and remember these without being *very comfortable* with the rest of the chest film first. For this reason, I will only present the cardiac anatomy you really need to know to make sense out of a chest x-ray. The left ventricle shadow is normally larger than the right. Remember also that the right ventricle is anterior to the left ventricle. As such, its shadow on the PA or AP chest x-ray is superimposed on that of the left ventricle. This is very important when looking for the proper placement of intracardiac lines, such as the tip of a temporary pacemaker.

The shadow of the heart on the chest film is called the *cardiac shadow* or *cardiac silhouette*. This shadow may or may *not* actually represent just the heart itself. For example, a pericardial effusion leads to enlargement of the the cardiac silhouette. And, the effusion would *not* be obvious from the plain chest x-ray... we'd need an echocardiogram to make that determination.

The edge to edge width (diameter) of the heart shadow at its widest part on the PA or AP film should normally be less than one-half the total intrathoracic diameter. If the diameter of the heart shadow is greater than this, there is radiographic evidence of cardiac enlargement. Remember that radiographic enlargement of the *cardiac shadow* does not necessarily correlate with anatomic hypertrophy as measured by EKG or on autopsy. Similarly, a small heart on chest x-ray does not necessarily correlate with anatomic cardiac hypoplasia.

> *REMEMBER* — **Radiographic enlargement of the *cardiac shadow* does not necessarily correlate with anatomic hypertrophy as measured by EKG or on autopsy.**

Positioning, especially on supine portable AP chest films, can lead to artifactual magnification, making the heart shadow appear larger than it really is. Increased lung volume makes the heart appear smaller by increasing the ratio of expanded lung to heart. The most common cause of a "small heart" on the chest x-ray is chronic obstructive pulmonary disease (COPD).

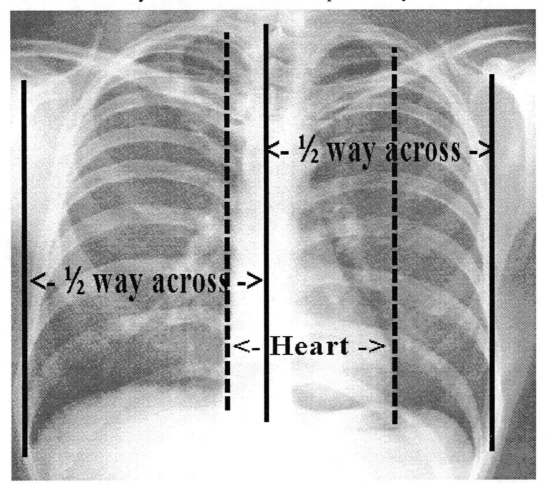

Normal Cardiac Diameter — the heart at its widest point should be less than ½ the distance across the chest at its widest point...

Figure C-4

Many patients with COPD actually have *enlarged hearts*. The lungs are overinflated due to air trapping. More x-rays pass through the fairly radiolucent lung, making the heart shadow appear smaller than it really is.

The hilar markings — The term "hilum" refers to the point of entry of blood vessels into an organ. So, the hilum of the lung is where the pulmonary arteries enter. On the normal upright chest x-ray the vascular markings passing from the mediastinum to the lungs are visible bilaterally. The right and left pulmonary arteries form a "hump" on each side of the film, and then branch into smaller vessels — the shadows of these smaller vessels form the hilar markings. On the left side, the heart shadow overlies some of these markings, but they should still be easily visible by "looking behind the heart" using a bright light ("hot light").

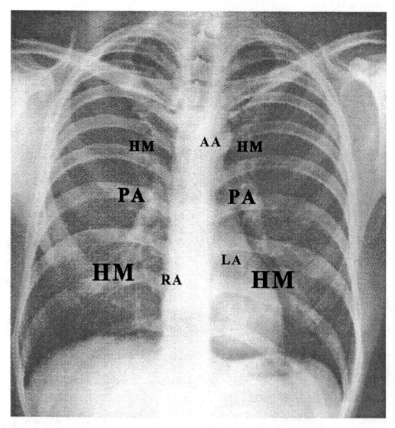

Pulmonary Arteries (PA) and Normal Hilar Markings (HM)

Figure C-5

Immediately below the pulmonary artery shadows on each side are the atria (RA, LA on Figure C-5). The aortic arch lies above the left pulmonary artery shadow (AA on Figure C-5).

REMEMBER — "Hot lights" actually *do* get quite warm and can melt the film if left on long enough!

Normally, in an upright film you see more hilar markings in the lower than in the upper portions of the chest. The reason is simple — in an upright patient, gravity tends to pull just enough of the vascular flow downward to make the inferior vessels more prominent than the superior ones. What about if we take an AP film with the patient supine? Will this effect still be present? No — the markings should be equal, upper and lower lobes, because the effect of gravity is now from anterior to posterior, not superior to inferior.

So, if you come across a chest film where the upper and lower vessels are equally prominent, what is the significance? If it's a supine film, this may be normal. On the other hand, if the patient is upright, then equal prominence of the upper lobe vessels is *abnormal*. Usually, it is an early sign of congestive heart failure — increased pressure in the pulmonary vessels counteracts the tendency of gravity to favor flow to the inferior portions of the lung. We'll talk more about CHF in a while...

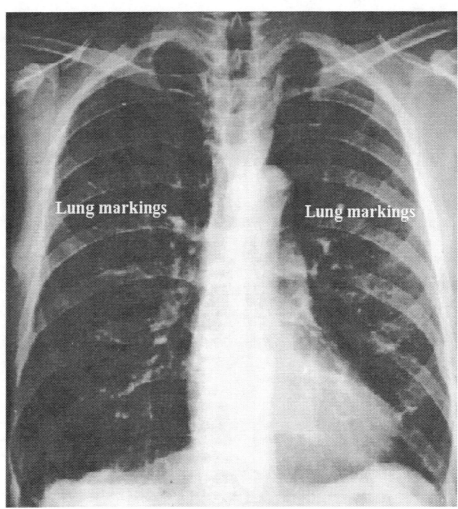

Figure C-6 — Normal lung markings

The lung markings — In addition to the hilar markings, you should be able to see lung markings throughout the lungs to the periphery. These markings consist of a combination of airways, vessels, and lung parenchyma and look like soft, streaky lines (Figure C-6). Occasionally, the x-ray beam passes through a vessel on end, leading to a nodular appearance in the midst of the lines. The easiest way to see these normal markings is to hot light the film. Absence of lung markings is usually abnormal.

The lateral chest film — Identification of structures is less precise on the lateral film. It is most helpful to pinpoint infiltrates and lesions. There are three normal "rules" for the lateral chest (Figure C-7):

- The diaphragm shadows should be clear.

- The shadow of the upper vertebrae is whiter than that of the lower vertebrae. Above, the film beam has to traverse not only the spine, but the shoulders and chest tissue. The resistance to passage of the beam is greater, so fewer x-rays hit the film, causing a whiter shadow. Lower down, the shoulders and chest are out of

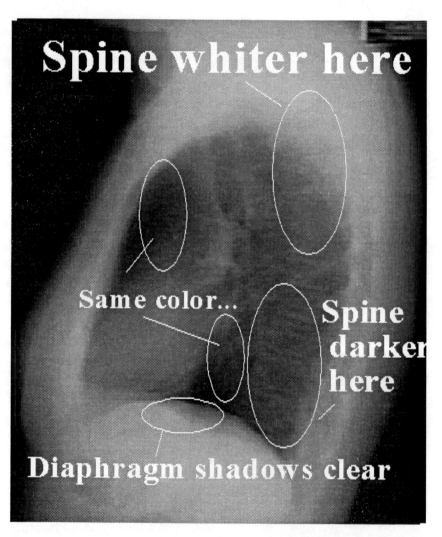

Figure C-7 — Normal Lateral Chest Film

the way, allowing more of the beam through to hit the film. The result? A darker lower vertebral shadow.

- The retrosternal and retrocardiac spaces should both be the same "color," and are both normally dark.

If any of these three rules is violated, there is fluid in the lungs, the pleural cavity, or both. Typically, the presence of fluid obliterates at least two out of three of these normal shadows.

AN EASY WAY TO MAKE SENSE OF JUST ABOUT ANY CHEST FILM

Fortunately, most everything you'll ever need to know about a chest x-ray can be summarized in three simple rules:

- **"We are symmetrical"** — Except that the right hemidiaphragm is slightly higher than the left, that the left heart shadow is more prominent than the right, and that the aortic knob causes a left-sided prominence *not* visible on the right, the normal AP or PA chest x-ray is symmetrical. The first thing you should do when you look at a chest film is move your eyes back and forth, left to right, as you scan down the film. Ask yourself if it is symmetrical. If there is a lack of symmetry, *stop* and describe why — what are you seeing?

    For example, a large radiopaque mass may be present at the left hilum (Figure C-8). As you scan, you realize that "we are not symmetrical." Why? — a "big hunker" (nonmedical for "mass") in the left hilum that isn't there on the right. Don't try and make a premature guess at a diagnosis — identify the asymmetry, describe it (e.g., left hilar white hunker), and then think about *what* it could represent. By itself, the lack of symmetry will reveal nearly 85% of chest x-ray abnormalities worth seeing. *Always* use the second rule as well, regardless of what you see on the "symmetry scan."

- **"Lung markings go all the way out"** — Start centrally and follow the pulmonary markings, described above, to be sure that they go *all the way to the edge* of the film.

Many times, the hot light will help you see them. Don't just look in one area — make it a *habit* to start in the middle of the heart and systematically

> **REMEMBER — If there aren't any lung markings, there isn't any lung!**

look radially from center to edge along the entire lung field. The beauty of this somewhat "compulsive behavior" is that it forces you look at the *entire* lung field. By doing this, you'll pick up small lesions, as well as

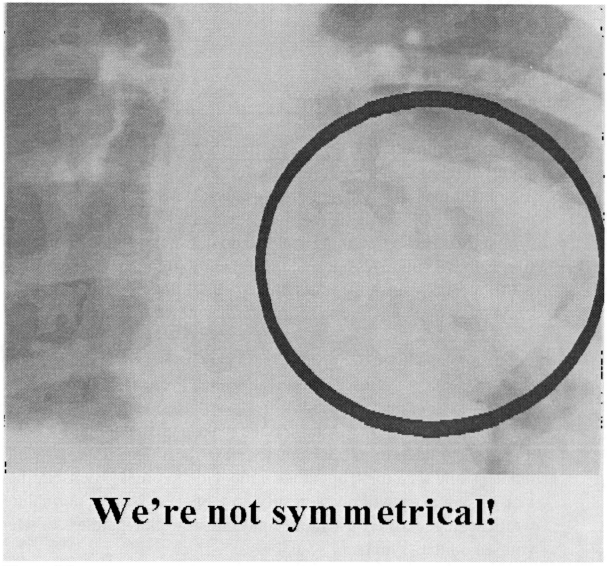

We're not symmetrical!

Figure C-8

peripheral small pneumothoraces usually missed using the symmetry rule, by itself. And, if there are no lung markings, there isn't any lung — it's either collapsed or absent (the surgeons have visited...). *Always* use this second rule even if you see an obvious abnormality using rule number one!

- **"Bones are smooth; when they're not, they're broken!"** — We'll use this rule for every single bone in the body. Look at the cortex of the ribs, clavicles, and sternum — it should be smooth. When there is a break in the cortex, suspect a fracture (Figure C-9).

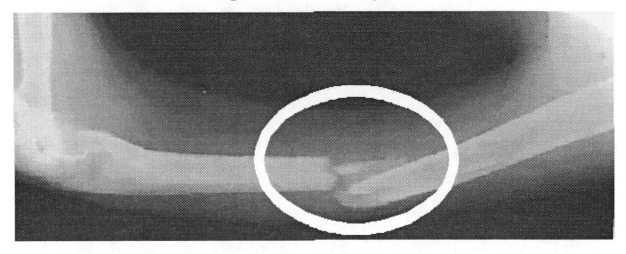

Bones are smooth; when they're not, they're broken

Figure C-9

ABNORMAL AIR SHADOWS

After properly identifying the film and making sure the quality is acceptable, use the "IQAWBF" acronym to evaluate the third item, "air" (gas) shadows. In the chest x-ray, we don't normally see a "pure" air shadow, except the stomach "gas" bubble in the upright film. Remember, the lungs contain not only air-filled alveoli, but tissue as well. So, the air-filled lungs should never appear completely dark. Rather, we see an intermediate density, best appreciated by looking at lung markings and making sure that they go all the way to the edge. We'll go over the details of a few important conditions to make sure you understand why the films look the way they do. Then, go back to the rules above ("we are symmetrical," etc.) — you'll find that just about every time, using them will point out the problem!

Pneumothorax — Pneumothorax is an abnormal collection of air in the pleural cavity. Think of the lung and pleura as two balloons, one inside the other (Figure C-10A). Most of us remember seeing these fancy balloons at a circus. Visualize the inside balloon as the lung and the outside one as the pleural cavity. Normally, the outside balloon is nearly completely collapsed, with the visceral and parietal pleura close to each other, and a small amount of pleural fluid in between. Remember, the pleural space is actually a "potential space," and the outer balloon (pleural space) only fills with fluid or air under abnormal conditions.

When air accumulates in the outside balloon, the inside balloon shrinks to a variable degree depending on the size of the pneumothorax. Let's start out with a large pneumothorax (Figure C-10B). If lots of air accumulates within the outer balloon (pleural space), the inside balloon (lung) collapses significantly. If you think of the lung as a sponge, it becomes compressed and more dense. The increase in density is reflected on x-ray as an *increase* in radiopacity. Fewer x-rays pass through to hit the film, resulting in

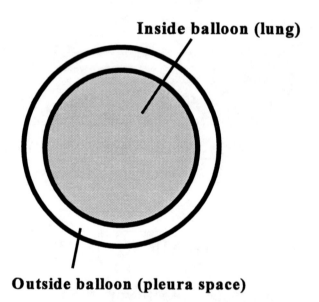

Inside balloon (lung)

Outside balloon (pleura space)

Think of the lung and pleura as two "circus balloons," one inside the other...

Figure C-10A

a *whiter* than usual shadow. So, we have the dense inner balloon (collapsed lung), the air-filled outer balloon (pleural space), and the surrounding ribs.

Imagine an x-ray beam passing through various places on the affected side. If it travels between the interspaces and hits the collapsed lung, the beam is attenuated (partially blocked). Since not many x-rays travel through to hit the film, the shadow of the collapsed lung is whitish, indicating its relative radiopacity. Where the beam hits the ribs, it is also attenuated, resulting in a radiopaque (whitish) shadow on the film. Often, the collapsed lung is more radiodense than the ribs and appears whiter on the film.

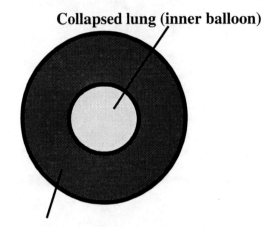

Collapsed lung (inner balloon)

Air-filled pleural space (outer balloon)

Large Pneumothorax

Figure C-10B

Consider what happens when the beam travels between the interspaces and through only the outside air-filled balloon. Since air is very radiolucent, most of the beam gets through, striking the film plate. The shadow of the outside balloon (air-filled pleural cavity) is dark because many x-ray beams have hit the film. If the x-ray beam traverses at the junction of the inner and outer balloons, it "sees" an area where two materials of very different radiodensities meet. Based on the rules above, you expect to see what? Of course, a sharp border ("BILL!"). With a large pneumothorax, the findings are usually fairly obvious, even without searching for a border. On the other hand, a small pneumothorax may not be so obvious. Finding the border between the air-filled pleura and the partially collapsed lung becomes essential.

Envision in your mind what the x-ray of a large pneumothorax *must* look like. Then look at the actual x-ray film. Make certain you *understand* why the film looks the way it does. Once you're comfortable with the appearance of a large pneumothorax based on the reasoning I've outlined above, we can apply the basic rules of the chest and make it even easier...

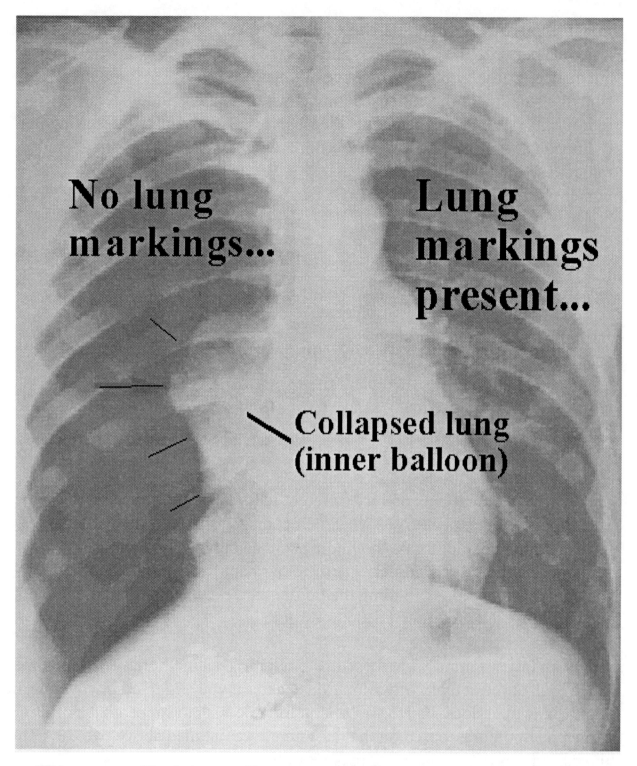

Figure C-11 — Large right pneumothorax

The first rule of the chest is "we are symmetrical." Look at the chest film of a large pneumothorax (Figures C-11, C-12). Is it symmetrical? No way — one side is white, the other is mostly dark. And the mostly-dark side also has a large radiopaque shadow near the hilum. Wait — don't jump to conclusions yet — I know *you know* that this film represents a large pneumothorax. But, let's pretend for a minute that you don't. The beauty of the rules is that they help you to figure out what might be going on *without* lots of sophisticated tools. If the film isn't symmetrical, describe to yourself why not — exactly what do you see? Now, let's go to the second rule.

The second rule of the chest is "lung markings go all the way out." If you follow the lung markings from the central region to the periphery of the normal side, they go all the way out. Guess what — if there aren't any lung markings, there ain't no lung!! So, our choice as to what might be going on becomes relatively limited... What about the asymmetrical side? You might be able to see lung markings within the collapsed lung, but they go no further. In this example the bones are smooth, but always look for abnormalities such as a fractured rib that may cause the underlying pneumothorax.

> **REMEMBER — If there aren't any lung markings, there ain't no lung!**

Now, put this all together... one side (left) is normal. The other side (right) "features" a radiopaque mass near the hilum with no lung markings beyond. The remainder of the hemithorax shows rib shadows with underlying dark areas and no lung markings within. What

> **REMEMBER — A large pneumothorax is usually easy to pick out because the chest won't be symmetrical.**

causes dark shadows on the x-ray? Either air (gas) or fat — since it's highly unlikely that the patient has a "lipothorax," the most likely explanation is that air (gas) has accumulated in the pleural space (outside balloon). Most likely

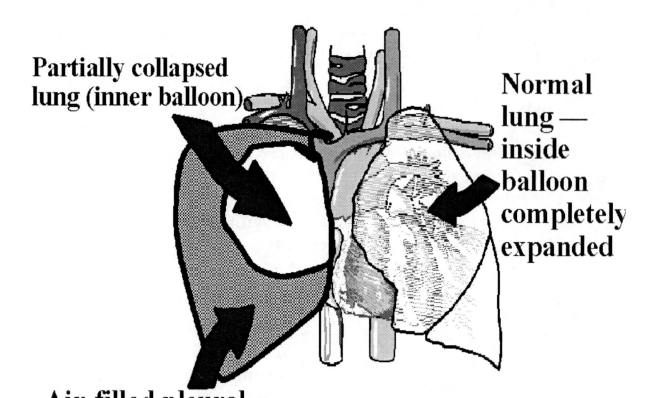

Partially collapsed lung (inner balloon)

Normal lung — inside balloon completely expanded

Air-filled pleural sac (outer balloon)

Figure C-12 — Right pneumothorax

"diagnosis" — large right pneumothorax. Review this logic in your mind until you are completely comfortable with how I reached this conclusion. Use the three basic rules to help you.

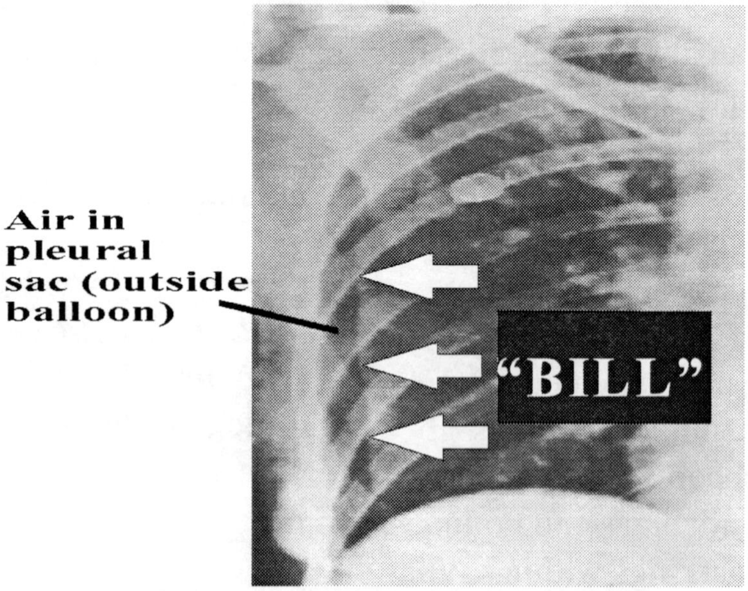

Air in pleural sac (outside balloon)

"BILL"

Figure C-13 — Small right pneumothorax

In smaller pneumothoraces (Figure 13), the asymmetry may not be as obvious. Always look for lung markings radiating to the periphery throughout all portions of the chest film. Absence of markings, especially if there is an interface, suggests a pneumothorax. The other major advantage of following the markings all the way out throughout the chest is that your eyes are directed across the entire lung field. You're much more likely to see small shadows or other abnormalities this way.

REMEMBER — If the lung markings suddenly stop at an interface, with dark shadows distal to the line, think of pneumothorax.

Overlapping skin folds can occasionally mimic the air-lung interface of a pneumothorax on chest x-ray. The clue is that, in the absence of pneumothorax, lung markings continue to be visible all the way to the periphery of the chest. If in doubt, repeat the film. Another normal shadow that may mimic pneumothorax is the scapular border. Again, look for lung markings extending beyond the line.

A final trick to pick up smaller pneumothoraces — if you strongly suspect the diagnosis on clinical grounds, get both an inspiratory *and* an expiratory chest film. Sometimes, a very small pneumothorax is hard to see on the typical inspiratory film. A film taken in expiration changes the ratio of lung to pleural space, and makes the pneumothorax far more obvious.

In a **tension pneumothorax**, the collapsed lung is shifted towards the opposite side. This produces respiratory and hemodynamic compromise. Sometimes, you can see the shift on the chest x-ray. A tension pneumothorax may still be present despite a lack of x-ray findings. The pneumothorax may not be that big. It is the *physiologic effects* of the pneumothorax, not its size, that matter

REMEMBER — It is the physiologic effects of a pneumothorax, not its size, that matter clinically.

clinically. Rely on the *clinical findings* to suspect a tension pneumothorax — if you wait for the x-ray, both you and the patient will likely suffer!

If air collects in the mediastinum, the condition is called **pneumomediastinum**. Air appears as linear radiolucent streaks or dots within the mediastinum (Figure C-14). Sometimes, they overlie the heart as well. An accompanying pneumothorax may or may not be present. Pneumomediastinum occurs in association with trauma, asthma, or rupture of the esophagus. It has also been reported during childbirth because of repeated episodes of increased abdominal pressure and airway rupture following contractions.

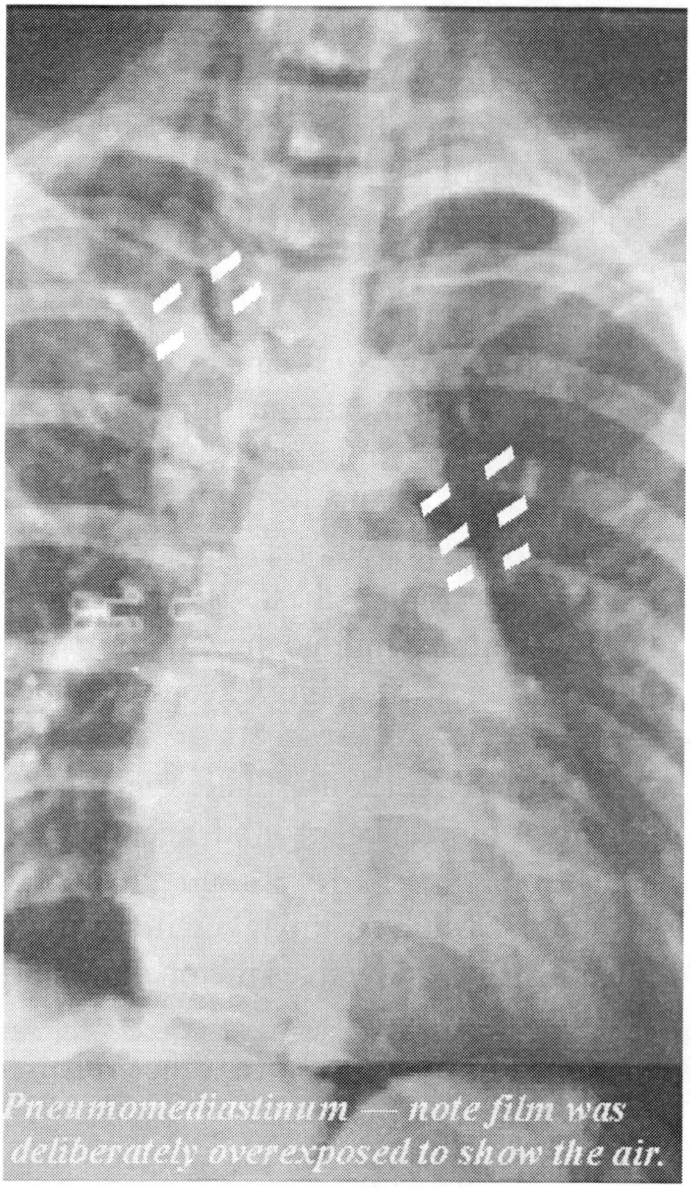

The simple way to recognize pneumomediastinum is to look for "black dots" over the mediastinum. If you see these, they must represent something that is radiolucent (lots of x-rays hit the film). Our choices are air

Pneumomediastinum — note film was deliberately overexposed to show the air.

Figure C-14

> *REMEMBER* — **Always look for abnormal air shadows about the mediastinum and over the heart. If you find pneumomediastinum, be sure to exclude concomitant pneumothorax.**

and fat — logic dictates, in this case, that air is the most likely candidate. Don't jump to the conclusion, though, that *all* "black dots" represent air (gas). In other areas of the body (e.g., the elbow) these may represent normal (or abnormal) fat shadows.

Ruptured diaphragm — post-traumatic rupture of the diaphragm is most common on the left side. Any of the abdominal organs may herniate into the

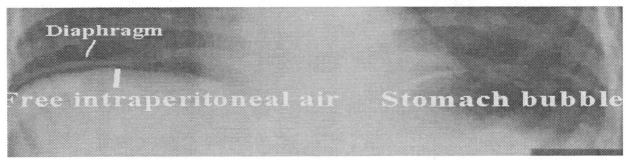

Diaphragm

Free intraperitoneal air   Stomach bubble

Figure C-15

pleural cavity. The result is collapse of some lung tissue, as well as the presence of abnormal structures in the chest. This is a *difficult* diagnosis to make in many cases. Sometimes, the only sign is a paper-thin diaphragm, indicating free intraperitoneal "air" (gas) [Figure C-15]. Other times, the herniated abdominal contents cause a vague radiopaque shadow in the left side of the lower left hemithorax. Only rarely are you lucky

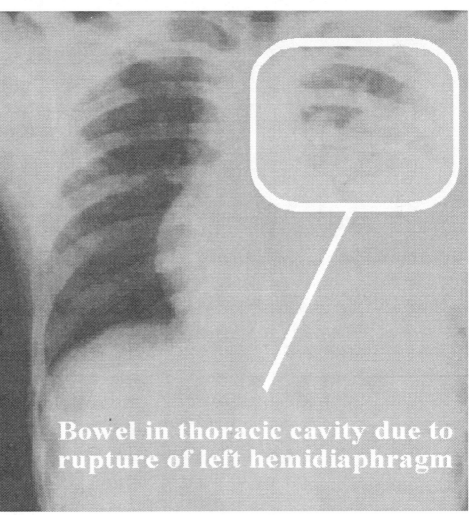

Bowel in thoracic cavity due to rupture of left hemidiaphragm

Figure C-16

enough to be able to make out typical bowel shadows in the chest (Figure C-16)! Obviously, if present, this is highly suggestive of a diaphragmatic hernia. Even though we've not talked about the abdomen yet, think about it — you can probably predict exactly what you'll see... Bowel contains gas, so there would be dark shadows; depending on the position of the patient, you might also be able to see air-fluid levels from material moving through the intestine.

The "rules of the chest" will lead you to the abnormalities, even if you have never heard of a ruptured diaphragm. Look for symmetry — abdominal contents in the chest will create extra radiopaque densities, making the film asymmetrical. Lung markings will usually be absent over the area of herniated abdominal contents as well. As for bones, look for fractures of the lower ribs on the affected side (usually the left).

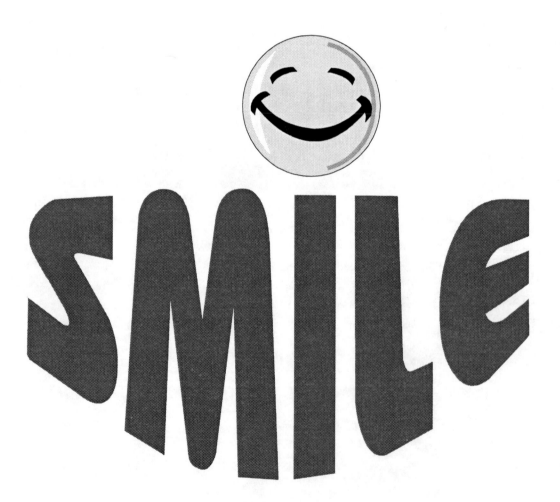

Asthma/COPD — the common denominator in both severe asthma and chronic obstructive pulmonary disease (COPD) is resistance to expiratory air flow. Air is trapped in the lungs, resulting in abnormal hyperinflation. As the lungs hyperinflate, the diaphragm is pushed inferiorly, and appears flattened on the x-ray. As the lungs grow "bigger" due to hyperinflation, there is relatively more air in the chest cavity through which x-rays can pass. The result? The lungs appear darker and larger than in the normal film. Due to lung hyperexpansion, the relative size of the heart shadow appears to shrink, and the hilar markings appear to be suddenly "cut-off." Anatomically speaking, of course, this is not the case — true, the lungs *have* become hyperinflated and the diaphragm flattened, but the heart and hilar vessels usually remain the same size (Figure C-17).

In some cases (e.g., cor pulmonale), the heart is anatomically *enlarged*. It doesn't usually appear abnormally large, at least by radiogaphic criteria, because the lung shadows are bigger due to hyperinflation. Thus, the COPD or asthmatic's x-ray is a great example of the *lack of correlation* between anatomic heart size and radiographic cardiac enlargement as measured on the

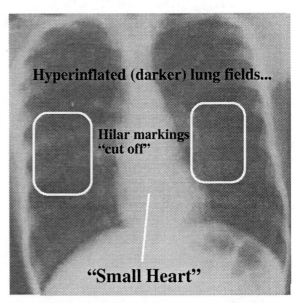

Hyperinflated (darker) lung fields...

Hilar markings "cut off"

"Small Heart"

Results of air trapping from asthma or COPD...
Figure C-17

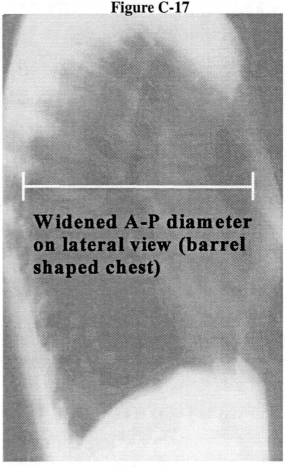

Widened A-P diameter on lateral view (barrel shaped chest)

Figure C-18

chest x-ray. That's precisely why we use the term "cardiac silhouette" or "cardiac shadow" instead of just "heart." In the lateral view, the chest will appear to be "barrel-shaped" due to hyperinflation (air-trapping) [Figure C-18].

Generally, there is little if any correlation between a patient's pulmonary function (FEV1, vital capacity, peak expiratory flow) and the appearance of the chest x-ray. In fact, I hope that you don't really need an x-ray to diagnose an exacerbation of COPD or asthma. The only indication for a chest film in asthma is when the patient fails to respond to conventional therapy (inhaled bronchodilators, aminophylline, steroids). In this case, you want to rule out a pneumothorax, pneumomediastinum (dark air

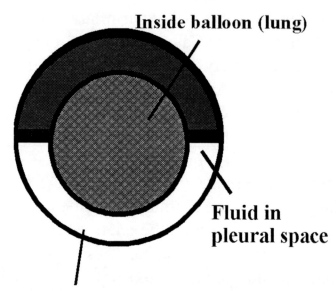

Inside balloon (lung)

Fluid in pleural space

Outside balloon (pleura space)

Pleural Effusion and the Two-Balloon Model

Figure C-19

shadows over the mediastinal area), or an infiltrate (see below). In COPD, some health care providers routinely obtain a chest film — I'm not one of them. Remember, the findings often only corroborate that an abnormality exists and don't correlate with disease severity. I get a film if the patient doesn't improve with "conventional" therapy, looking for the same abnormalities as outlined earlier for asthma.

ABNORMAL WATER (FLUID) SHADOWS

Fluid shadows appear as radiopaque densities on the chest x-ray. Again, the basic rules prove very helpful.

Pleural effusion — Pleural effusions are abnormal collections of fluid in the pleural cavity. Since these shadows have the same radiographic density as fluid in the lungs (infiltrates), it is sometimes difficult to tell whether fluid is in the pleura space, the lungs, or both. A couple of simple tricks will help. Again, use the two balloon model we discussed above. This time, though, we'll put liquid rather than air into the outside (pleural) balloon (Figure C-19). In addition, it helps to think of a single plastic bag, partially filled with liquid, to represent the pleural space and effusion.

In an upright view, pleural fluid forms an air-fluid level, or a meniscus in the outer balloon.

When the patient moves, so does the fluid...

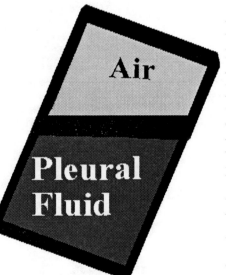

Figure C-20

Imagine your fluid-filled plastic bag as you hold it. When you tilt it to one side or the other, what happens? The fluid moves, doesn't it? And the very same thing happens within the outside balloon or pleural cavity. If the patient is moved, the fluid shifts position — and this usually occurs within a few minutes (Figure C-20), unless there is scar tissue in the way (loculated pleural effusion). Fluid within the lungs themselves doesn't usually shift — if it does (as is sometimes the case in CHF), the process requires *hours* rather than the five or ten minutes it takes for pleural fluid to move.

Now, look at your fluid-filled bag from the side. What do you see? A level or **meniscus** forms at the junction of air and liquid. If you see a whitish shadow on the chest film with a level on top, it's probably a pleural effusion. Of course, you usually can't say much about the *underlying lung* since it's invisible. By moving the patient, though, you shift the fluid and can then discern the underlying lung to see if it is normal or not.

An important point to remember is that without additional information, it's usually impossible to tell the *type* of fluid you are seeing. For this reason, I've coined the term "fluothorax," meaning liquid in the pleural cavity (pleural effusion) of unknown type. It could be blood (hemothorax), tumor, pus (empyema), extravasated total parenteral nutrition (TPN) fluid (lawsuit), or any other liquid — you just can't tell by the film alone. Don't try to make a diagnosis when the required information

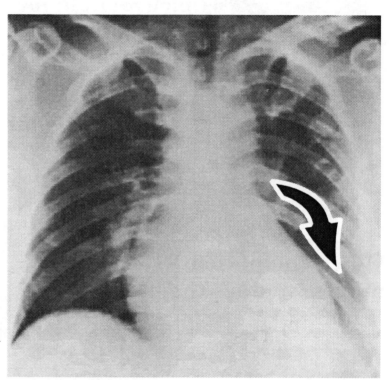

Blunting of left costophrenic angle suggests pleural effusion...

Figure C-21

isn't there. On the other hand, if I told you that the patient had just been run over by a dump truck, and also had a bunch of broken ribs, you'd be reasonable in suspecting that the fluid is blood — a hemothorax.

On the AP or PA chest film the first sign of a pleural effusion is blunting of the costophrenic angle on one or both sides (Figure C-21). Think of this as someone's taking a "white highlighter" and filling in the edge. Though some texts refer to minimal blunting of the costophrenic angle as indicative of a "small pleural effusion," this is not anatomically correct. To understand why, we need to look at the lateral chest film.

> **REMEMBER — The first sign of pleural effusion on the AP or PA chest film is blunting of the costophrenic angle.**

The diaphragm is curved and is higher anteriorly than posteriorly. In fact, the posterior diaphragm dips downward, outlining the **posterior sulcus** or posterior costophrenic angle. Envision the x-ray beam coming through on the AP or PA film. Unless the posterior sulcus contains a material of unusual radiodensity, the beam passes through and "sees nothing." It is, however, attenuated when it passes through the liver and diaphragm on the right, and the spleen, stomach, and diaphragm on the left. Make certain you are convinced why this "posterior triangle" is normally "invisible" on the standard AP or PA film.

The costophrenic angle, as seen on the PA or AP film, correlates anatomically with the top of the triangle. Thus, for the angle to be blunted, the entire posterior sulcus must be filled in first. The only time you will see blunting of the costophrenic angle is when the fluid has filled the posterior sulcus, and started to

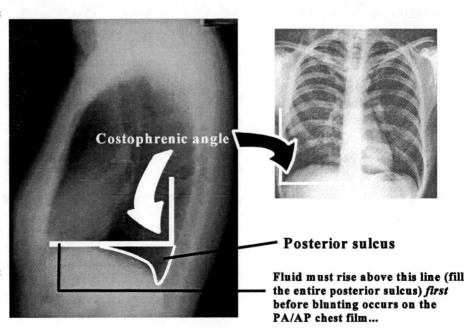

Costophrenic angle

Posterior sulcus

Fluid must rise above this line (fill the entire posterior sulcus) *first* before blunting occurs on the PA/AP chest film...

Figure C-22

"flow over the brim of the dam" which is the top line of the triangle. Translation — even minimal blunting of the costophrenic angle indicates that the posterior sulcus *must* have been filled in first. So a "small effusion" on AP or PA films actually represents the volume of the "triangle" *plus* the volume of fluid visible in the blunted angle. Typically, the volume of the posterior triangle is between 250 and 500 cc, depending on the patient. Granted, some pleural effusions may be much

REMEMBER — A "small pleural effusion" seen on the AP or PA films is really at least 250 - 500 cc in size.

larger, but a 500 cc effusion is far from insignificant! So, when you see blunting of the costophrenic angle, it suggests a pleural effusion of *at least* 250 - 500 cc (Figure C-22).

As the pleural effusion increases in volume, what do you expect to see on the PA or AP film? The white shadow gets bigger and bigger, as if someone had filled in the darker spaces with a "white highlighter." Usually, the effusion obscures the heart border — why? Since both the heart and pleural effusion are fluid densities, there is no "BILL." So, another hint as to the presence of abnormal fluid (either in the pleural cavity or in the lungs) is obliteration of the

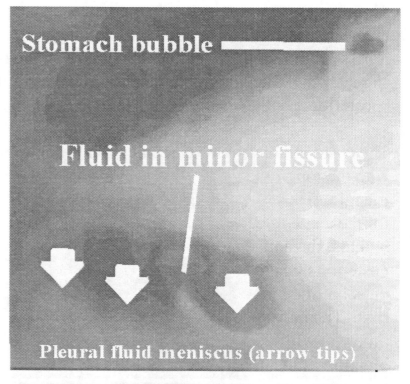

Right lateral decubitus film...

Figure C-23

cardiac border. The same thing occurs with the border of the diaphragm shadow.

Since the shadow of pleural fluid "whites out" all the other markings, it is difficult to tell if the lung markings go all the way out, or if there is also fluid in the lung tissues (infiltrate). The best way to figure this out is to move the patient, causing the pleural fluid to shift and allowing you to get a better view of the lungs. The most common film for this purpose is the **lateral decubitus** view. The patient lies with the fluid-containing side down (right lateral decubitus or left lateral decubitus), causing the fluid to shift. The fluid forms a meniscus (fluid level), and you are able to visualize the lung above the line. In a standard upright or supine view, much of this lung tissue would normally be covered by pleural fluid and difficult to see (Figure C-23). Though the film should be marked, verify that the correct side is down (against the film) by observing the heart shadow and stomach bubble, both left-sided structures (assuming that the patient doesn't have total *situs inversus*!).

Imagine how a pleural effusion would appear in different views. Let's assume you see a rather large right-sided effusion, meniscus included, on the PA view (Figure C-24). What would the lateral view look like? How about if we laid the patient down and took a supine chest film? Think about it...

From the lateral view, again you'd expect to see a large whitish shadow, often with a meniscus (Figure C-25). Not difficult, is it? As the patient lies supine, the fluid flows to the dorsal part of the pleural cavity — convince yourself by again turning the bag of fluid on its side. In the supine view, the x-

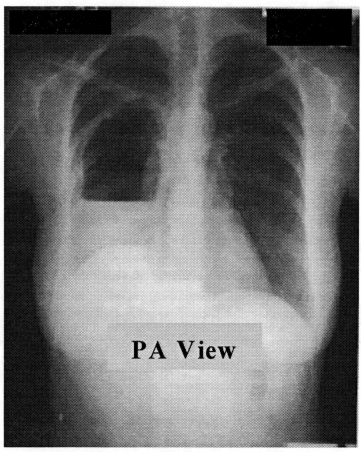

PA View

Figure C-24 — Right pleural effusion

ray beam passes through fluid in all areas of the affected hemithorax. The resulting shadow is totally white, or a "white out" of the involved hemithorax.

Now, let's look at the same concept in a slightly different way. Assume that you obtain a supine film on a patient and see a white-out of the left hemithorax (see Figure C-26). Since I know you're the curious type, you'll want to know if the fluid is in the lungs, in the pleural cavity, or both, right? What is the best way to do this? — move the patient and see if the fluid moves. If you sit the patient up, pleural fluid should move and form a meniscus. Similarly, you'd expect the same thing if we obtained a left lateral decubitus film.

Sometimes, air *and* fluid enter the pleural cavity. The resultant "aerofluothorax" causes collapse of at least some underlying lung tissue. It's easy to picture this if you go back to our two balloon model (Figure C-27). Imagine the outside balloon (pleural cavity) partially filled with water, the remainder with air. The air lies on top of the fluid and at the point

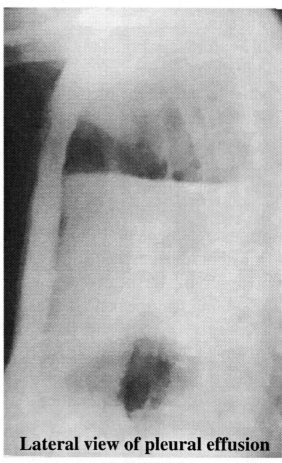

Lateral view of pleural effusion

Figure C-25

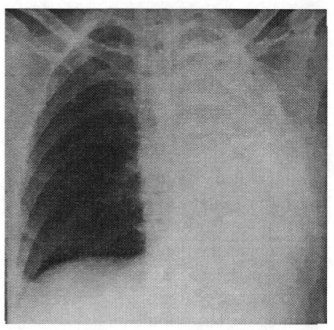

"White-out" of left hemithorax — where is the fluid?

Figure C-26

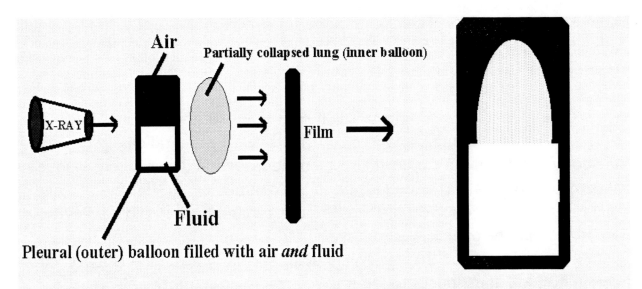

Diagram of "aerofluothorax" (hemopneumothorax). Film shows overlying air and fluid level in outer balloon with shadow of collapsed lung above; little, if any, of collapsed lung will be visible through the fluid.

Figure C-27

they meet there is an interface. In your mind, layer this balloon between the ribcage and the partially collapsed lung (inner balloon). You then expect to see two radiopaque shadows — one representing the partially collapsed lung, the other the fluid. There is also a dark area, representing air in the pleural cavity, above the fluid, but devoid of lung markings due to lung collapse. This is a common appearance for a hemopneumothorax (blood and air in the pleural cavity) but remember you can only make the diagnosis with additional information. Just the appearance of the x-ray, *by itself*, does not allow you to reach this conclusion!

All of the above findings should easily be seen if you follow the three basic rules of the chest. The lack of symmetry is apparent when one side of the film is normal "color," while the other has two abnormal white shadows, and an area of black, not

> *REMEMBER* — **Pleural fluid changes position in response to gravity. If you're not sure that a shadow represents a pleural effusion or a lung infiltrate, move the patient. A pleural effusion will shift within 10-15 minutes, while an infiltrate stays much the same.**

seen on the other side. Then, look at the lung markings — they don't go out all the way, stopping at the border of the dark area and the whitish (radiopaque) shadow.

Lack of lung markings peripheral (distal) to a new radiopaque area suggests what? A collapsed lung... and you confirm air in the pleural cavity by seeing the border and radiolucent air shadow. In addition, the layered radiopaque shadow is almost always due to fluid in the pleural cavity. Putting one and one together, you conclude: collapsed lung, air and fluid in pleural cavity. Knowing that the patient was run over by a moving van, you strongly suspect hemopneumothorax on the involved side. Especially if trauma is involved, be certain to look at the bones to see if they are smooth or not.

A lung infiltrate may be present along with a pleural effusion. Usually, you can still see shifts in the effusion by moving the patient. Sometimes, it is impossible to tell the difference between a diffuse

> *REMEMBER* — **Blunting of the costophrenic angle suggests the presence of pleural fluid.**

infiltrate and a large effusion. The most helpful clue is that pleural effusion is more likely than lung infiltrate to blunt the costophrenic angle.

Pericardial effusion — Fluid in the pericardial space is called pericardial effusion. Fluid accumulation results in enlargement of the heart shadow on chest x-ray. When there are at least 200 cc of pericardial fluid, the heart may take on a "water bottle" appearance. It is difficult to tell the difference between a pericardial effusion and cardiac enlargement on plain x-rays. An echocardiogram usually gives a quick answer.

Infiltrates — An x-ray shadow of fluid in the lung is an infiltrate. Technically speaking, there are two types — interstitial and alveolar. An **interstitial infiltrate** is fluid located in the connective tissue

> *REMEMBER* — **On the x-ray, fluid in the lungs is called an infiltrate. Fluid in the pleural cavity is called a pleural effusion.**

between the alveoli and other smaller airways (interstitial tissue). On the other hand, an **alveolar infiltrate** represents fluid *within* the alveoli. Sometimes, an infiltrate involves both the interstitium and the alveoli. On x-ray, interstitial infiltrates appear as streaky white shadows while alveolar infiltrates look more diffuse or fluffy, much like

> *REMEMBER* — It is difficult to tell what type of fluid is in the lungs just by looking at the x-ray. Blood, pus, lymph, and serum may all look alike.

"snowballs" at times. Though the difference between interstitial and alveolar infiltrates is important in some people's minds, most of us use the more descriptive terms below. The reason is communication — do you really know what I mean by an "alveolar" or a "mixed" infiltrate? Isn't it easier to picture what I mean by a "diffuse, streaky infiltrate?"

As I said earlier, descriptive terms for infiltrate make it easier to communicate what we see to our colleagues. The most common types of infiltrates are (Figure C-28):

- A **streaky infiltrate** appears as linear bands of increased density ("white streakies"). The lines represent fluid in the interstitial tissue of the lungs. Thicker streaky infiltrates are referred to as **plate-like** infiltrates. It is impossible to differentiate plate-like infiltrates from plate-like **atelectasis**, small sections of collapsed lung, on a single film.

- A **patchy infiltrate** looks like scattered patches of increased fluffy density ("white fluffies"). Think of a target that has had several snowballs thrown at it. This type of infiltrate represents filling of the alveoli with fluid.

> *REMEMBER* — It's more important that you be able to recognize an infiltrate in the first place than to classify it as streaky, patchy, diffuse, or a white-out.

- A **diffuse infiltrate** is an area of increased density involving a significant portion of one or both of the lung fields. Diffuse infiltrates may be streaky, patchy, or a combination of the two. When an infiltrate appears as though someone took a white paintbrush and "colored-in" an entire area, the infiltrate is often referred to as **confluent**.

•   A **white-out** is an infiltrate that involves all of one or both lung fields. It is a commonly-used term for a large, diffuse, and confluent infiltrate. When the infiltrate is this large, you cannot distinguish between a patchy and a streaky infiltrate.

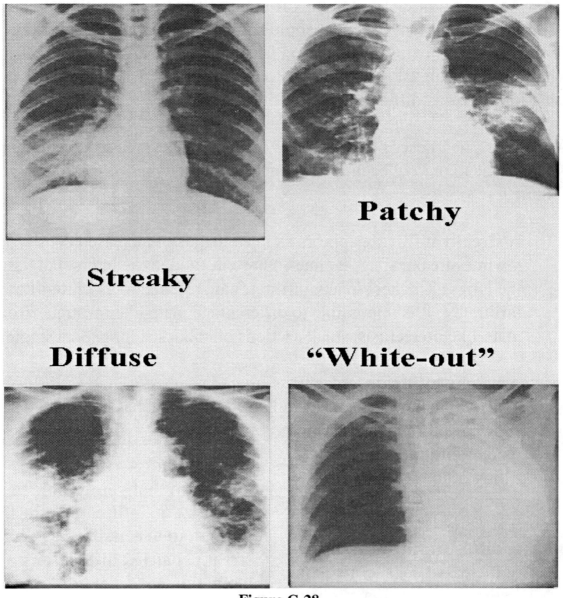

Figure C-28

Don't get ahead of yourself by looking at a film and immediately making a diagnosis, such as "this is an *obvious* infiltrate of community-acquired diplococcal pneumonia." Relying on the x-ray by itself is a poor way to make a diagnosis because a particular infiltrate (shadow) may be caused by many different things.

Look first for symmetry — if there's an infiltrate present, the film will usually be asymmetrical. Once you notice asymmetry, describe why — what do you see that leads to that conclusion? Is it a streaky white shadow, "snowballs," a diffuse white shadow? Is the pleural space involved as well or is there just fluid in the lungs (infiltrate)? Then, go to the second rule... by following the lung markings all the way out, the infiltrate should become obvious. After describing what you've found (e.g., diffuse infiltrate in the right upper lung field), then proceed to consider what may be going on. Add in other clinical information to formulate and narrow down a differential diagnosis.

> **REMEMBER — Use all available clinical data, not just the x-ray alone, to make a diagnosis.**

> **How to Look at a Chest X-Ray**
>
> - **Do you like what you see? Would you like to be the "proud owner" of that film?**
>
> - **Are we symmetrical? If not, *describe* what you see. Then...**
>
> - **Do lung markings radiate all the way out?**

Look at the film to your right (Figure C-29) — what do you see? Is it symmetrical? Sure doesn't look that way to me... the patient's left side is normal, but on the right side is a confluent white infiltrate. The costophrenic angles look sharp, ruling against effusion.

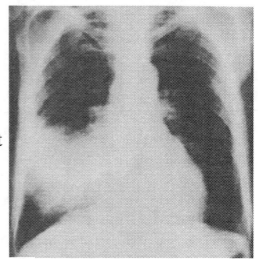

Figure C-29

Radiographically, it's possible to further pinpoint this and many other infiltrates. For infiltrate localization purposes, both lungs have essentially three lobes — the right and left lungs have upper and lower lobes (Figure C-30). The right lung has the middle lobe (RML), while the left lung has the lingula, technically part of the left upper lobe. The right

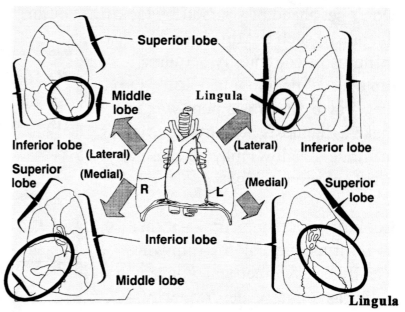

Figure C-30

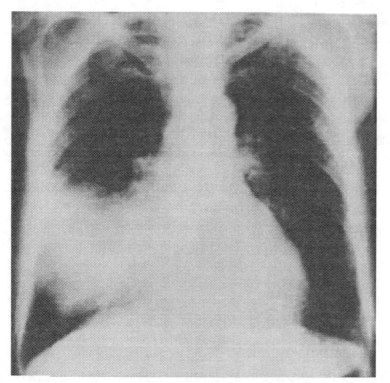

Right Middle Lobe Infiltrate (obliterates heart border)...

Figure C-31

middle lobe and the lingula on the left side are in roughly the same anatomic location, respectively, on each side of the chest — anterior to and right up against the heart.

Remember there is no interface between two objects of the same radiographic density. An infiltrate in either the right middle lobe or in the lingula will lead to a fluid shadow immediately against the fluid density of the heart. The result? The heart border is obliterated.

So a mid-lung field infiltrate on the right side that obliterates the right heart border is likely in the right middle lobe (Figures C-31, C-32). And, an infiltrate of the left mid-lung field that obliterates the left heart border is probably in the lingula.

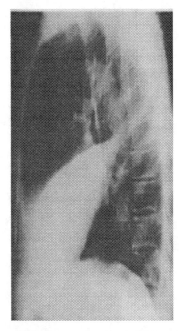

Lateral View — RML or Lingular Infiltrate

Figure C-32

Understand clearly in your mind *why* these infiltrates *have to* wipe out the heart border. Normally, you see the border because of the interface between air-filled lung and fluid-filled heart. When the right middle lobe or the lingula fill with fluid (infiltrate), the composition of the interface changes to a liquid-liquid border. And, when the substances are of the same radiographic density, there is *no* interface between them ("Bye-bye BILL!"). So, the affected heart border disappears. Always verify your suspicions, when possible, by a lateral view ("one view is always one view too few!)...

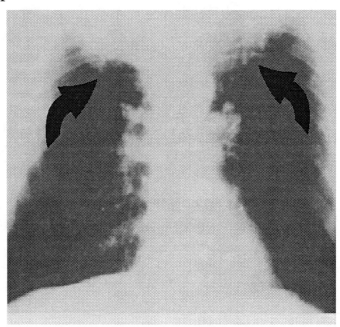

Figure C-33

Similarly a lower lobe infiltrate, on either side, usually obliterates the diaphragm shadow. The heart border remains visible because the lower lobes are posterior and the heart, anterior. Even when filled with fluid, a posterior infiltrate cannot abut against the heart to blur out its shadow. Upper lobe infiltrates may obliterate normal shadows in the upper mediastinum, but should *not* affect the heart border (Figure C-33).

The only conclusion you should reach when you first identify an infiltrate is that there is fluid in the lungs. As with pleural effusions, it is *nearly impossible* to determine the composition of the fluid from the film alone. Too often, people see an infiltrate and instinctively guess pneumonia! Look at the film below (Figure C-34). What do you see? Is it symmetrical? If not, why not? Describe how you reached your conclusions.

I suspect that by now, you've learned that the *wrong* thing to do is to shout out "pneumonia." What you should notice is that the chest is not symmetrical. The reason — a whitish fluffy infiltrate in the left side of the hemithorax.

Otherwise, the lung markings go all the way out, and the visible bones appear smooth. Note that the left heart border is intact (though somewhat difficult to see because the infiltrate has nearly the same density as the heart), but that the diaphragm shadow is obliterated. So, the infiltrate is probably in the left lower lobe. A lateral film would confirm your suspicions. At this point, the only thing that you can *safely conclude* is that there is a left lower lobe infiltrate. Though the

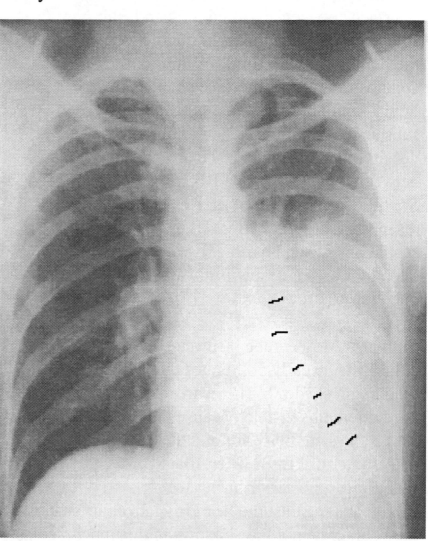

Figure C-34 — Left lower lobe infiltrate (note heart border is clear, but difficult to see because the infiltrate has a similar density...)

uninitiated might jump ahead and say that this is a film of "an obvious community-acquired diplococcal pneumonia," (which it is, by the way) — remember that there are several possible explanations for the appearance of this x-ray:

- If the patient is a 25 year old male presenting with cough, green sputum, fever, shaking chills, an elevated white blood cell count, and has extraneous breath sounds over the left side of the chest... the film is compatible with, but *not diagnostic for* pneumonia. Remember, pneumonia is a clinical diagnosis based on cough, sputum production, fever, white count, and physical findings of lung consolidation. Sometimes, the x-ray is negative. Go by the clinical findings and the patient's

  > *REMEMBER* —Don't try to conclude more than is "educationally sound, medically correct, and legally defensible"!

  appearance. Remember that one of the worst pneumonias, *pneumocystis carinii*, often presents with a *normal chest x-ray* in a hypoxic, short of breath patient. If the patient is a 66 year old male who presents with weight loss, massive axillary adenopathy, and a 200 pack-year smoking history... suspect *lung tumor*.

- If the patient is an 18 year old woman on birth control pills and presents with left-sided pleuritic chest pain, has tachypnea (RR=30), and a room air pO_2 of 30 mm Hg (normal > 80 mm Hg at sea level)... I'd think about a *pulmonary embolus* (PE) with subsequent *lung infarction*. An embolus, by itself, doesn't cause an infiltrate unless there has also been pulmonary infarction, which is uncommon. Though

  > *REMEMBER* — Many common entities may look exactly the same on a chest x-ray; don't rely on the x-ray alone to make a diagnosis.

many x-ray signs have been associated with embolism over the years, none are specific. Other than ruling out other causes of the patient's symptoms, the chest x-ray contributes little to the diagnosis of PE.

- If the patient is a 50 year old male involved in a motor vehicle accident who hit his left chest on the steering wheel... consider a *pulmonary contusion*.

- If the patient is a 34-year old woman with autoimmune disease, she could have *Goodpasture's Syndrome* with alveolar bleeding. The resulting shadow on the chest film would look the same as the patients' described above.

And, we could go on and on... All of the above conditions, as well as many more, lead to the accumulation of *fluid* in the lungs. On chest x-ray, the infiltrate *looks the same*. Don't rely on the x-ray by itself to make a diagnosis. Please, remember that the amount of information we get from an x-ray is limited. Don't try to conclude more than is "educationally sound, medically correct, and legally defensible"!

COMMON CONDITIONS THAT CAUSE INFILTRATES

The last thing I want you to do is jump to a "diagnostic conclusion." On the other hand, since I hope you'll use this book for reference later on, I felt inclined to include information about some common clinical situations for which you might obtain a chest x-ray and find an infiltrate.

Congestive heart failure — Congestive heart failure (CHF) occurs when the pumping capacity of the heart is impaired. The left ventricle is most commonly involved ("**left heart failure**"), though concomitant involvement of the right ventricle ("**right heart failure**") is being diagnosed more and more commonly. When the heart fails, two related series of events occur:

- The *muscle fibers stretch*, leading to cardiac enlargement or dilation. In chronic CHF there is both dilation and hypertrophy of muscle tissue. The basis for stretching of muscle fibers is **Starling's Law** — this "bird" recognized that to an extent, the contractility of a muscle is *increased* if it is stretched a bit prior to contraction. Thus, dilation is Mother Nature's way of increasing cardiac contractility. Sometimes it works, but with progressive disease, pumping efficacy continues to worsen despite increasing myocardial size.

> *REMEMBER* — The normal diameter of the heart shadow on the chest x-ray is less than one-half the distance from the lateral rib border to the middle of the thoracic vertebrae.

Normally, the heart shadow should be *less than one-half the intrathoracic diameter* (Figure C-35). As the heart dilates in the CHF patient, the shadow often gets larger than this, leading to radiographic evidence of cardiac enlargement (increased cardiac silhouette). Remember, as we

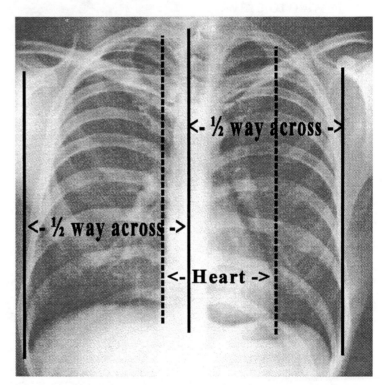

***Normal Cardiac Diameter* — the heart at its widest point should be less than ½ the distance across the chest at its widest point...**

Figure C-35

discussed earlier, that this finding does *not* necessarily correlate with anatomic or EKG hypertrophy. And don't forget that persons with cor pulmonale (predominantly right sided failure) may have cardiomegaly despite the x-ray appearance of a *smaller* heart due to air trapping and hyperinflation in the lungs.

- *Pressure increases in the pulmonary vessels*, leading to a predictable series of events. Remember that in a normal upright chest film more hilar vascular markings are seen in the *lower* than in the *upper* lobes due to gravity. In early CHF, increased pressure causes all of the pulmonary vessels to swell. In the upper lobe vessels, this elevation counteracts the tendency of gravity for more flow to be directed inferiorly. The effect —

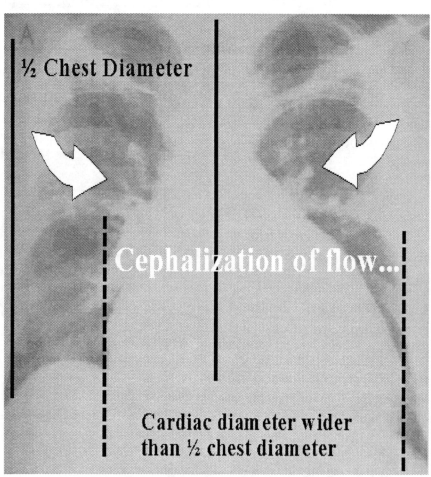

Figure C-36

increased vascular markings in the upper lobes. Thus, you'll see the upper and lower vessels looking pretty much the same — and this finding is distinctly *abnormal* in the upright film (Figure C-36). The formal name for this phenomenon is **cephalization** of flow or

redistribution of flow to the upper lobes. Some describe it as looking like **deer antlers**. So, if the vessels are equally visible in the upper and lower lobes in an upright chest x-ray, especially if the heart shadow is enlarged, we have pretty good evidence for early congestive heart failure. Some people also refer to Kerley lines — small horizontal lines at the lung periphery that indicate early interstitial fluid. Cephalization of flow is a *much more* reliable sign and is easier to see. Though others may disagree, I personally don't find Kerley lines very helpful.

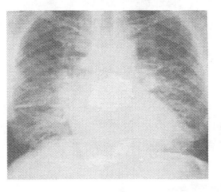 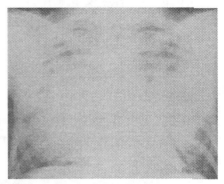

- As the pressures continue to increase, the swollen vessels begin to leak fluid into the interstitial tissues. This results in a haziness about the hilum, often referred to as the **butterfly appearance of the hilum** (Figure C-37).

"Butterfly Hilum"

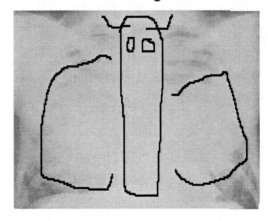

Figure C-37

- As fluid starts to fill in the alveoli, the butterfly starts to fill in, often with the appearance of scattered round, fluffy shadows, or a **snowball** appearance (Figure C-38). Combined with cardiac enlargement, this appearance is strongly suggestive of, *though not diagnostic for*, cardiogenic pulmonary edema (did you like my little "legal disclaimer"?).

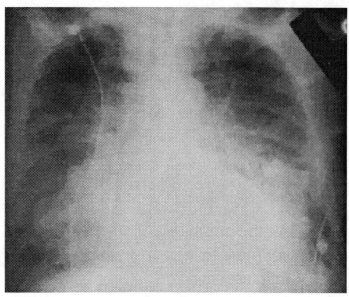

Figure C-38

Though it's always important to start off with the rules of the chest, the symmetry principle might not be as helpful here as in some other cases. Often the deer antlers, butterflies, and snowballs, as well as cardiac enlargement, are relatively *symmetrical*. So, you can conclude that the film is symmetrically *abnormal*!!

CLINICAL HINT — **There are no specific chest x-ray findings diagnostic for myocardial infarction. An initial film, however, is helpful as a baseline and to evaluate for the presence of CHF.**

Following the lung markings is also essential so you don't miss a small pneumothorax — especially common if the patient has been placed on positive pressure ventilation. Looking for markings also draws your eyes across the *entire* film so you don't miss a more subtle finding. By the way — many cardiac patients have easily visible radiopaque circles a few millimeters in diameter on the chest... any idea what they are? Read on for the answer (page CHEST-58).

CLINICAL HINT — **The most common cause of cardiomegaly and bilateral infiltrates is congestive heart failure.**

Noncardiogenic pulmonary edema — Noncardiogenic pulmonary edema is associated with a number of conditions. The primary underlying anatomic cause is increased permeability of the pulmonary blood vessels. The best-known type of noncardiogenic pulmonary edema is adult respiratory distress syndrome (ARDS). It is difficult to make the diagnosis of ARDS from a chest x-ray alone. Suspect ARDS when you cannot adequately oxygenate a patient with 100% FIO$_2$. The chest x-ray shows normal heart size, and bilateral diffuse infiltrates. In addition, there is no redistribution of blood flow to the upper lobes (Figure C-37). If the patient has a concomitant lung infection, there is no way to differentiate infiltrate due to fluid from the infection from infiltrate due to noncardiogenic pulmonary edema.

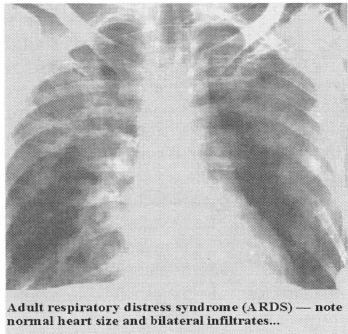

Adult respiratory distress syndrome (ARDS) — note normal heart size and bilateral infiltrates...

Figure C-39

Pneumonia — Pneumonia is an inflammation of the lungs caused by either infectious agents or irritants. It sometimes appears on the x-ray as an infiltrate. Different types of pneumonia have different appearances on x-ray. Your major responsibility is first to recognize that an infiltrate exists. You cannot make the diagnosis of a pneumonia from an x-ray film alone. The only thing you can safely say is that there is an infiltrate.

> *REMEMBER* — **ARDS is primarily a clinical diagnosis. The patient has a normal-sized heart and bilateral infiltrates, no cephalization of blood flow, and cannot be adequately oxygenated on 100% FIO$_2$.**

Often, there is a **lag time** of up to twenty-four hours between the appearance of clinical signs and symptoms, and the appearance of an infiltrate on x-ray due to pneumonia. At times, this lag may occur because the patient is dehydrated. If the patient has clinical findings suggesting lung consolidation, the most likely diagnosis (if all else fits) is pneumonia, *regardless* of what the chest film shows. The reverse of this phenomenon is common in patients with severe congestive heart failure. Even though the patient may get better within a few minutes of initial treatment, the chest film looks "sick" for up to another twenty-four hours. It takes that long for the accumulated pulmonary edema fluid to clear radiographically!

> *CLINICAL HINT* — The x-ray appearance of a lobar pneumonia is the same as that of a pulmonary infarction following pulmonary embolus. You can only make the diagnosis by knowing clinical information.

Pulmonary Embolism — Pulmonary embolism (PE), by itself, rarely results in any diagnostic x-ray findings. The most common chest x-ray in a patient with PE is a normal film. Other nonspecific findings include elevation of the diaphragm and pleural effusion on the involved side. If the involved lung tissue infarcts, which is uncommon, an infiltrate will form. This process takes several days to occur. Of course, with the x-ray alone you cannot differentiate pulmonary infarction from other causes of infiltrate.

> *REMEMBER* — The most common chest x-ray finding in a pulmonary embolism is a normal film.

Pulmonary Contusion — A pulmonary contusion is a bruise to the lung that occurs from trauma. It appears on the x-ray as an area of infiltrate, the size of which depends upon the amount of lung tissue involved. The infiltrate represents bleeding into the alveoli and the interstitial tissue. Overlying rib fractures may or may not be present. The infiltrate from a pulmonary contusion looks the same on the x-ray as does the infiltrate from a pneumonia. Without clinical information, it is impossible to make the correct diagnosis.

> *REMEMBER* — **It is impossible to make the diagnosis of pulmonary contusion based on the chest x-ray alone. Use a combination of clinical information and x-ray findings.**

Aortic trauma — Traumatic rupture of the aorta is associated with a high mortality. 95% of patients die at the scene; the remaining 5% of persons form a hematoma at the rupture site (Figure C-40). This hematoma ultimately ruptures, though the time period until rupture ranges from minutes to years. Most of these contained hematomas will rupture within one or two hours. If we can identify high-risk patients and get them to the operating room, potentially life-saving surgery may be performed.

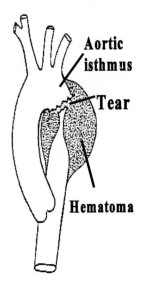

Figure C-40

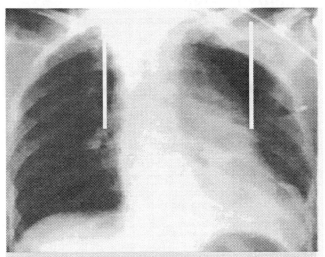

Widening of mediastinum due to aortic trauma...

Figure C-41

The most common location of rupture is at the aortic isthmus, distal to the takeoff of the left subclavian artery from the aortic arch. The most frequent chest x-ray finding is

> *REMEMBER* — **AP/PA chest x-ray findings associated with rupture of the aorta include widening of the mediastinum, left-sided pleural effusion, obliteration of the aortic knob, and fractures of ribs 1-3.**

widening of the mediastinum (Figure C-41). On an erect PA chest x-ray, the maximum normal width of the mediastinum in an adult is 8 cm. There are, however, no widely accepted criteria

> **REMEMBER** — Widening of the mediastinum in a trauma patient is due to rupture of the aorta until proven otherwise.

> **CLINICAL HINT** — Maintain a high index of suspicion for aortic injury. If there are any clinical or x-ray suggestions of the diagnosis, obtain an aortogram. An unstable patient needs to go directly to the operating room. An aortogram or chest CT scan is unnecessary.

for AP views. Normally, you should not see much other than the vertebrae above the level of the aortic arch. If you see an increase in shadows, consider the possibility of a traumatic aortic aneurysm. Sometimes you will also see left-sided pleural effusion, obliteration of the aortic knob, or associated fracture of ribs 1-3. Of course, a normal chest film *does not* completely exclude aortic injury.

ABNORMAL BONES (TRAUMA)

For completeness' sake, it's always important to look over the main bones seen on the AP or PA chest film — clavicles, ribs, sternum, and scapulae. There are no tricks to

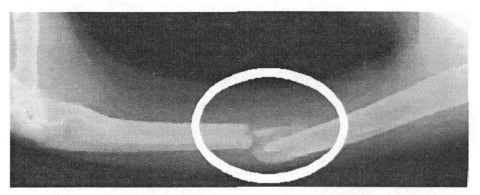

Bones are smooth; when they're not, they're broken

Figure C-42

making sense out of chest bone fractures, or any other fractures for that matter! Bones are smooth — if they're *not* smooth, they're broken (Figure C-42). Follow the outline of each bone, and make sure that the cortex is smooth. Breaks in the cortex suggest a fracture.

Rib fractures — The most commonly injured of the chest bones are the ribs. Rib fracture is often *not* visible on the chest film. In fact, it is one of *three* commonly missed fractures. The other two are navicular fracture of the wrist and stress fracture of the foot (primarily the tarsals and metatarsals). If you clinically suspect a rib fracture (history of trauma, point tenderness over the area), it's best to treat the patient as though a fracture were present, whether visible on the x-ray or not. Always remember to look for other associated trauma (e.g., pneumothorax). If you need to confirm the presence or absence of a fracture (such as in a workers' compensation case), either get a bone scan (which should "light up" in the region of an acute fracture) or obtain a film two weeks later to look for callus formation (healing).

> *REMEMBER* — **If at least five ribs are fractured or if at least three ribs are fractured in two different places, a flail chest is present.**

Due to their anatomic position, the first three ribs are well-protected. Injury requires a significant amount of chest trauma. Fracture of any of these ribs may be associated with severe underlying injury, such as aortic rupture.

> *REMEMBER* — **Assume that a patient with fractures of ribs 1-3 has a severe underlying injury until convinced otherwise.**

Isolated fractures of ribs 4 to 10 are not usually dangerous for the patient. But, fracture fragments can occasionally puncture nearby tissues, causing severe problems:

- Pleura — pneumothorax
- Liver — liver laceration
- Spleen — splenic laceration
- Major blood vessels — significant bleeding

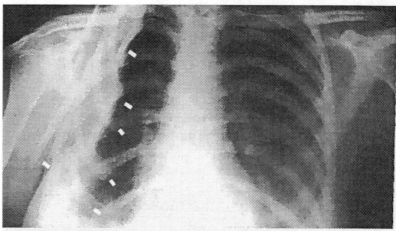

R. sided flail chest due to multiple rib fractures...

Figure C-43

Multiple rib fractures may lead to ineffective movement of the chest wall. If the injury is severe enough, the fractured segment may actually move in a direction *opposite* to the rest of the chest wall during breathing (**paradoxical breathing**). This condition is known as a **flail chest** (Figure C-43).

Sternal and scapular fractures —
Sternal and scapular fractures, by themselves, are painful but not dangerous. Note, however, that to fracture either of these relatively thick and well-protected bones requires *massive trauma*. Always look for associated injuries such as cardiac or pulmonary contusion, ruptured spleen or liver, and great vessel injury. In fact, *make a habit of always looking for underlying injuries whenever a patient has suffered enough trauma to fracture a bone — regardless of which one.*

> *REMEMBER* — **Multiple rib fractures lead to flail chest. The injured area moves in the opposite direction as the normal chest wall. This abnormal movement leads to a marked decrease in the effectiveness of breathing.**

Metastatic disease — Cancerous lesions cause *localized (often discrete)* changes in bony density versus **osteoporosis** which causes a diffuse decrease in density, produces a generalized "darker" appearance of affected bone. The ribs are rarely affected — far more commonly are the spine, pelvis, hips, and long bones of the lower extremities.

Different types of metastatic tumors cause different lesions — either osteolytic or osteoblastic. **Osteolytic** lesions destroy the normal bone matrix, resulting in areas of *decreased* radiographic density. **Osteoblastic** lesions create overgrowth of abnormal bone, leading to *increased* density. Normally, the bone density (degree of radiopacity or radiolucency) should be homogenous. Isolated changes in the density suggest tumor involvement. It may be difficult to tell if you are looking at a primary tumor or at a

> *REMEMBER* — **Bony lesions of the ribs are most likely due to metastatic tumor.**

metastatic lesion. Primary bone tumors of the ribs are very unusual. Bony lesions of the ribs are most likely due to metastatic disease. Sometimes, a bone scan is required to detect bony metastases.

FUNNY LOOKING THINGS

The most common "normal" funny-looking things are the nipple shadows. It's easy to reshoot the film using radiopaque nipple markers to be sure. Don't make the all too common mistake of thinking an early lung tumor is just a nipple shadow! Comparison to a patient's old films may prove invaluable in more ways than one! There are numerous funny-looking things that are *not* part of one's normal anatomy. Sometimes, we obtain x-rays to determine the position of one of these (e.g., an endotracheal tube). Other times, funny-looking shadows indicate underlying pathology (e.g., a lung mass) and must not be missed.

Tubes — Chest x-ray is a helpful way to determine *endotracheal (ET) tube* position, especially if the tube is placed in too far. The proper location for the tip of an ET tube is three to six cm above the carina — the point at which the trachea branches off into right and left mainstem bronchi (Figure C-44). Remember, using the carina to locate the tip of the ET tube *assumes* that the tube is within the trachea. X-ray is *not* the best tool to determine whether a tube is actually in the esophagus or in the trachea. They only help in deciding if an *intra-tracheal* tube is down far enough, or down too far.

> *REMEMBER* — X-rays are *not* the best tool to determine whether a tube is actually in the esophagus or in the trachea. They only help in deciding if an intra-tracheal tube is down far enough, or down too far.

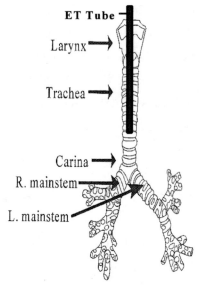

Figure C-44

There is only one way to determine accurately *where the carina is* on an x-ray — and that is actually to see it. Some sources report that you can count ribs or vertebrae to approximate the location of the carina. True occasionally, but these methods rely on a statistical bell curve. If the patient isn't in the middle of the curve, you're wrong — sometimes *dead wrong*! If you're looking for ET position and can't see the carina by hot-lighting the film, repeat the film until you can see it!

If the tube seems to take a C-shape turn to the patient's right, it is almost always in the right mainstem bronchus, but you should verify this by seeing the carina. An ET tube that is inserted too far down leads to inadequate ventilation to the rest of the lung fields. Conversely, if the tube isn't far enough in, patient neck movement can easily result in inadvertent extubation.
Compare the films below (Figure C-45, Figure C-46) — are the ET tubes in

the correct position? Can you see the carina? Are there any other obvious abnormalities seen on your "quick-scan" of the film? Do any of the films need to be repeated — if so, why? See the captions for the answers.

Chest tubes are placed into the pleural cavity to drain abnormal collections of fluid and/or air. The location of a tube depends on its desired purpose. Following trauma, tubes are usually placed in the third or fourth interspace at the midaxillary line. The tube should lie medial to the inner rib margin, well within the chest cavity. Remember that the AP or PA chest x-ray tells you nothing about the anterior-posterior orientation of the tip. Always get a lateral view as well to confirm good placement. Most chest tubes have a thin radiopaque line along their length that shows up on x-ray. Breaks in the line occur at the suction ports.

Intra-aortic balloons or intra-aortic balloon pumps (IABP) are placed percutaneously via the femoral artery to improve coronary artery perfusion. The tip should lie immediately distal to the takeoff of the left subclavian artery from the aortic arch (Figure C-

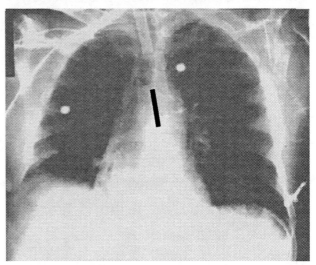

REMEMBER — If you can't see the carina the proper response to the question "is the tube in the right place," is: "I don't know because I can't see the carina!"

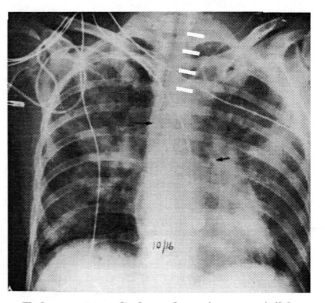

Figure C-45: tube in good position (line marks carina)

Tube appears C-shaped; carina *not* visible; tube probably down right mainstem... **REPEAT FILM!**

Figure C-46

47). Though the actual location is often confirmed by contrast dye during tube placement, the tip should lie below the medial end of the clavicle on the left side.

Lines — *Central venous pressure (CVP) monitoring lines*, more commonly known as *central lines*, are inserted for a variety of reasons. Central lines are often inserted via a peripheral arm vein to administer out of hospital therapy (e.g., antibiotics, chemotherapy, total parenteral nutrition). These are called *percutaneously inserted central lines* (PIC lines). Regardless of the intended purpose for the line, it should appear as a radiopaque "funny-looking thing" with the tip just above the right atrium (Figure C-47). If the tip passes into and perforates the heart, it may lead to cardiac tamponade.

> *REMEMBER* — **The tip of the CVP line must be in an intrathoracic position to accurately record the central venous pressure. It should, therefore, lie distal to the anterior first rib. Two common complications of CVP line insertion are pneumothorax and pleural effusion.**

> *REMEMBER* — **Always obtain a chest x-ray after placing a central line. Evaluate the position of the line and rule out complications, such as pneumothorax or pleural effusion.**

Most clinicians routinely obtain a chest x-ray after insertion of a central line. Evaluate the position of the line and survey for intrathoracic complications such as pneumothorax and pleural effusion. A patient who develops a new pleural effusion immediately after a central line has been placed could have hemorrhage or extravasation of fluid from the punctured vein.

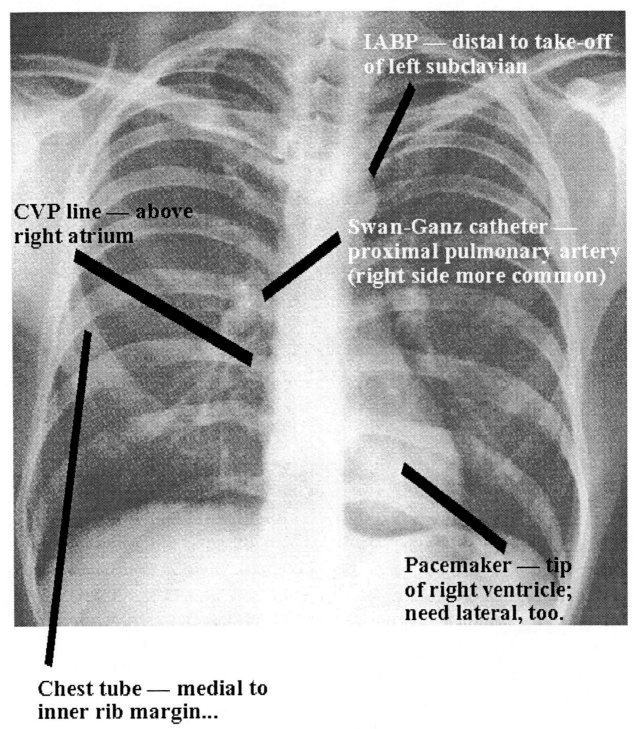

IABP — distal to take-off of left subclavian

CVP line — above right atrium

Swan-Ganz catheter — proximal pulmonary artery (right side more common)

Pacemaker — tip of right ventricle; need lateral, too.

Chest tube — medial to inner rib margin...

Figure C-47

Pulmonary artery flow-directed catheters, more commonly known as *Swan-Ganz catheters*, are placed via a central vein. After reaching the vena cava, the tip passes through the right atrium into the anteriorly-located right ventricle. From here, the catheter usually takes a posterior and rightward turn, ending up in the right pulmonary artery. Occasionally, it turns to the left, and lies in the left pulmonary artery. When the balloon is not inflated, the catheter tip should lie in the proximal pulmonary artery (right *or* left). On chest x-ray, this corresponds to just about the edge of the main hilar vessels (Figure C-47). A catheter that is out too far gives inaccurate readings and increases the risk of pulmonary artery rupture. If the catheter tip is not advanced far enough into the proximal pulmonary artery, inaccurate readings result. In addition, there is a great risk of the tip's slipping back into the right ventricle, causing ventricular tachycardia and cardiac arrest.

Pacers and leads — One of the most common funny-looking objects we see is the ***EKG monitoring lead***. Due to differences among leads and in patient positioning, they may appear simply as radiopaque densities, or have a more complex appearance. Either way, a very radiopaque funny-looking thing on the periphery of the chest is likely to be an EKG lead, especially if it's attached to a wire (Figure C-48).

There are many different types of ***intracardiac pacemakers***. Most rely on a set of electrodes placed either surgically or transvenously into the right ventricle and sometimes the right atrium. An emergency temporary pacemaker usually has only one lead wire. Permanent pacers have at least

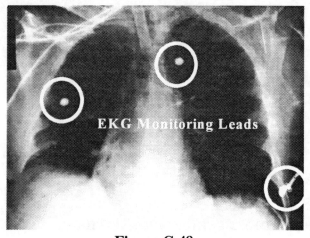

Figure C-48

> ***CLINICAL HINT*** — **Up to 20% of permanent pacer electrodes change position. Of these, a small number will perforate the heart. Suspect this complication when the tip of the electrode projects beyond the border of the myocardium or when the cardiac shadow rapidly enlarges (tamponade).**

two, sometimes more. Remember that the right ventricle is located anterior to the left ventricle. On the PA or AP chest film, it is impossible to determine whether the pacing electrode is anterior or posterior in the ventricle. It may even have penetrated the anterior right ventricular wall and, other than clinical presentation, appear completely normal on the PA or AP film. Always obtain a lateral chest film (Figure C-49) as well to confirm pacing electrode placement. In addition to the electrode(s), implanted pacemakers almost always show up on plain chest x-rays.

Automated implantable defibrillators (AID) consist of an implanted electrical pulse generator that contains various electronic components and three electrodes. One electrode is positioned in the superior vena cava. The second electrode is a flexible patch that covers the apex of the heart. These two electrodes sense the patient's electrocardiogram and serve as the defibrillation electrodes. A third electrode is placed in the right ventricle. This electrode records the EKG signal needed to synchronize with the R wave and determine the heart rate. At times, though, the AID is implanted in the upper abdominal wall and is not visible on the chest x-ray.

Masses — Round radiopaque shadows of various sizes are frequently seen on the chest x-

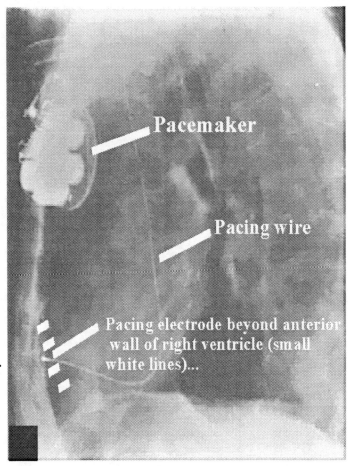

Permanent cardiac pacemaker

Figure C-49

ray. Many times, the smaller ones represent a blood vessel "on end" causing the appearance of a round mass (Figure C-50). Anytime you are uncertain as to whether a shadow represents a blood vessel or an abnormal mass, obtain additional films and perhaps other studies (e.g., CT scan) to help out. Round, radiopaque densities seen on the chest film are often called **coin lesions** because they resemble a coin — similar size, very whitish in color, and relatively sharp edges (Figure C-51). It is *nearly*

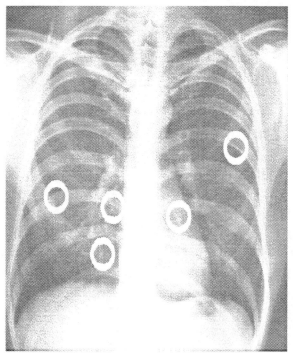

White circles surround normal shadows of blood vessels on end; remember the x-ray beam's path must travel down their entire length, not just across, causing the increase in density.

Figure C-50

impossible to make a diagnosis by looking at the film, by itself. On the other hand, you must identify any unusual radiopacity that is present. Causes of these lesions range from tuberculosis to pleural tumor. Again, the rules of the chest should come in handy.

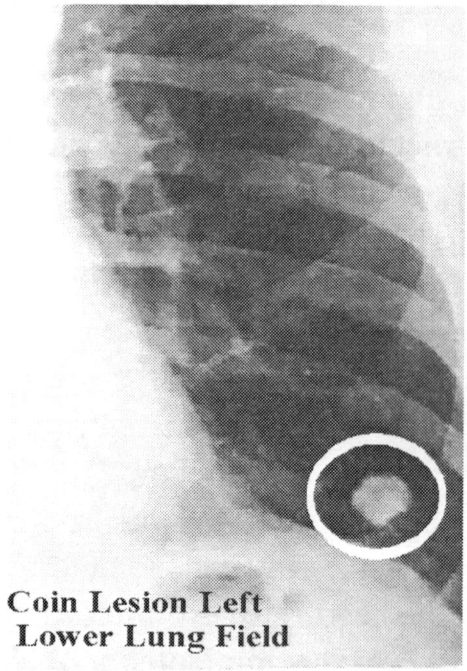

Coin Lesion Left Lower Lung Field

Figure C-51

Look at the film below (Figure C-52) and describe what you see. Is it symmetrical? Of course not — there is a white "hunk" in the right lung field that is conspicuously absent on the left side. Now, this one isn't real subtle, but if you missed this "hunkoma" using the rule of symmetry, you should definitely see it by following the markings to the edge. In this case, the bones are smooth. Again, the system comes through! More properly speaking, you might identify the abnormality as a large radiopaque coin lesion, or a radiopaque nodule. Either way — nodule, coin, or hunker — if you call the film "normal," you blew it! Once you've identified the lesion, it is relatively easy to formulate a list of possible causes. Throw in some clinical information and you're well on your way to a differential diagnosis!

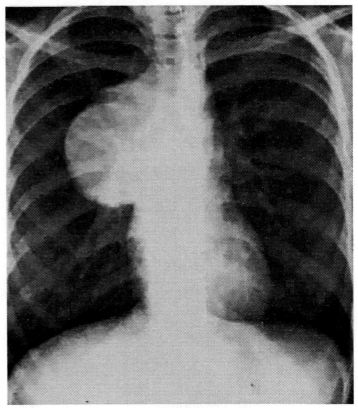

Figure C-52

Often mass lesions are asymmetrical. On occasion, abnormalities are symmetrical. A common example is bilateral hilar adenopathy from granulomatous disease such as sarcoidosis. Though it's impossible to actually make a diagnosis, you can easily identify the excess hilar opacity on both sides. This often represents hilar lymph node enlargement (lymphadenopathy) and sarcoid is a very common cause (Figure C-53).

Foreign bodies — Foreign bodies may be injected, inserted, aspirated, inhaled, or shot into a person. There are as many possible x-ray appearances as there are foreign bodies. The cardinal rule is to notice that one is present, then proceed to figure out what it is. The most common sign of a foreign body on chest x-ray is *seeing the shadow of a foreign body*. Sounds simple, doesn't it? Sometimes, it's more subtle, especially in children. If you suspect a nonradiopaque foreign body, get a chest film during both inspiration and expiration. A ball-valve effect causing hyperinflation of the involved side may become obvious on the expiratory film (what "color" would the affected side appear?). By the way, a great clinical trick is to give a bronchodilator — if wheezing only clears on one side of the lungs, there is a high likelihood of an intrabronchial foreign body in the still-noisy side. Remember that additional views are often needed to pinpoint and identify accurately a radiopaque foreign body. Sometimes, endoscopy or contrast x-ray studies may be required.

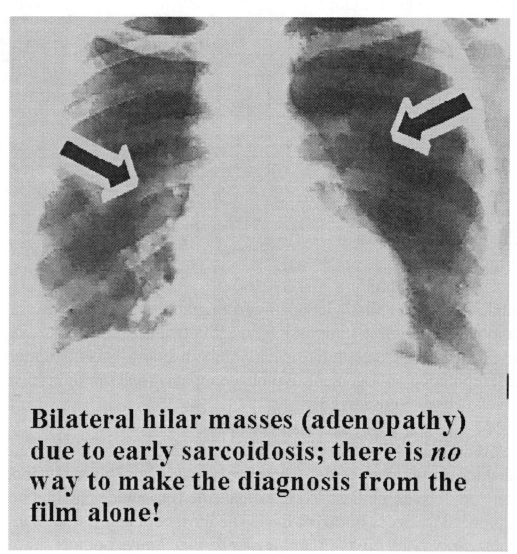

Bilateral hilar masses (adenopathy) due to early sarcoidosis; there is *no* way to make the diagnosis from the film alone!

Figure C-53

SUMMARY — Rules of the Chest

In the normal chest:

- Think of a tree.
- The right hemidiaphragm should be 1-2 cm higher than the left.
- The diaphragm should never be paper thin — if it is, there's abnormal air within (the peritoneal cavity).
- The costophrenic angles should be sharp and clear.
- The cardiac diameter is normally less than one-half the intrathoracic diameter.
- Hilar vessels are normally more prominent in the lower than the upper lobes in an upright film.
- Lung markings should be visible all the way to the periphery.

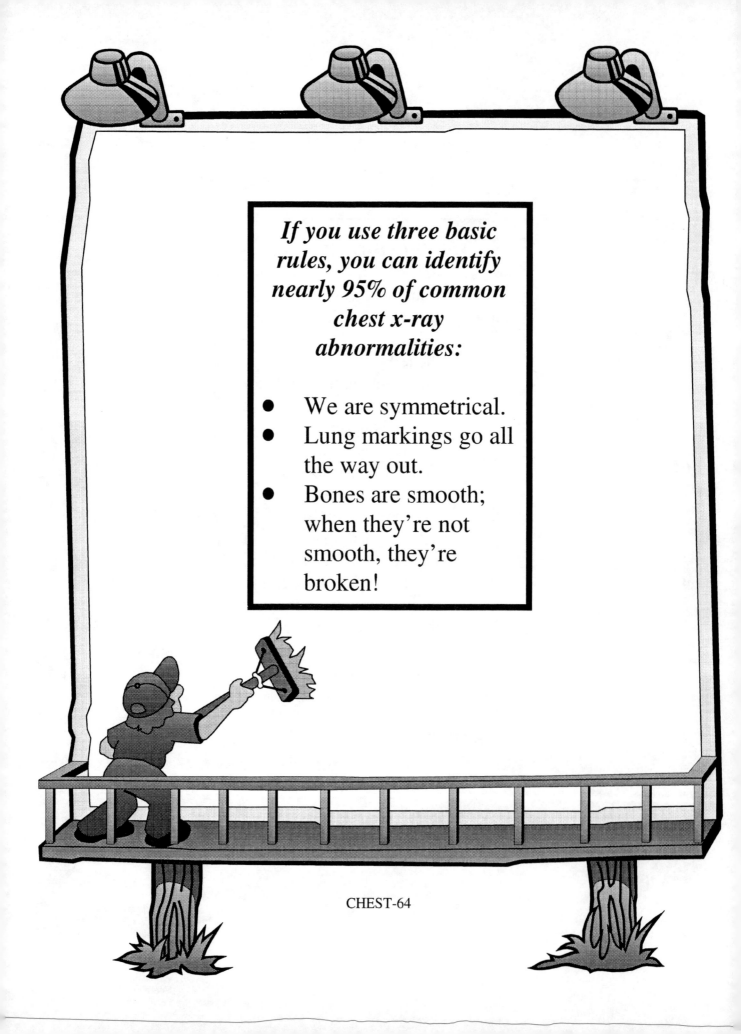

If you use three basic rules, you can identify nearly 95% of common chest x-ray abnormalities:

- We are symmetrical.
- Lung markings go all the way out.
- Bones are smooth; when they're not smooth, they're broken!

Think of the pleural cavity and the lung as one balloon within another.

Air in the pleural cavity ("outer balloon") is a pneumothorax.

Fluid in the pleural cavity ("outer balloon") is a pleural effusion; fluid in the lungs is an infiltrate.

Regarding abnormal air shadows:

- The physiologic effects of a pneumothorax, not its size, matter clinically.
- Always look for abnormal air shadows ("black spots") about the mediastinum and over the heart. If you find pneumomediastinum, be sure to exclude concomitant pneumothorax.
- Bowel loops in the chest suggest rupture of the diaphragm.
- A chest x-ray is most helpful in the asthmatic who is not improving with conventional therapy.
- A chest x-ray in COPD is most helpful when it reveals a complication, such as pneumothorax or pneumonia.

Regarding abnormal water shadows:

- Fluid has the same radiographic density whether it is blood, lymph, pus, or serum. You cannot distinguish simply by looking at the x-ray.
- Abnormal fluid collections in the pleural cavity ("outside balloon") are pleural effusions. Abnormal fluid accumulations in the lung tissue itself ("inside balloon") are infiltrates.
- The earliest sign of a pleural effusion is blunting of the costophrenic angle. Remember that 250 - 500 cc of fluid must be present in the posterior sulcus for even minimal blunting to appear on the PA/AP view.
- Pleural fluid changes position in response to gravity. If you're not sure if a shadow represents a pleural effusion or a lung infiltrate, change the patient's position. A pleural effusion will shift within 10-15 minutes, while an infiltrate stays much the same.
- It is more important that you be able to recognize an infiltrate in the first place than to classify it as streaky, patchy, diffuse, or a white-out.
- Use all available clinical data, not just the x-ray alone, to make a diagnosis.
- ARDS is primarily a clinical diagnosis. The patient has a normal-sized heart and bilateral infiltrates, no cephalization of blood flow, and cannot be adequately oxygenated on 100% FIO_2.
- It is impossible to make the diagnosis of pulmonary contusion based on the chest x-ray alone. Use a combination of clinical information and x-ray findings.
- Widening of the mediastinum in a trauma patient is due to rupture of the aorta until proven otherwise.

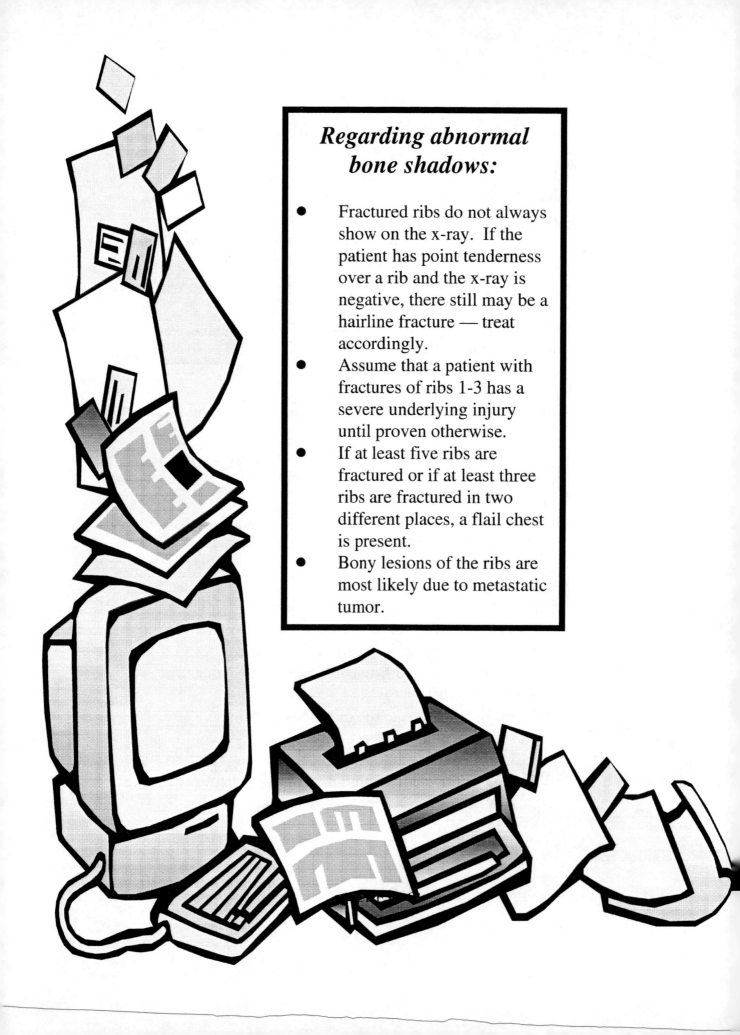

Regarding abnormal bone shadows:

- Fractured ribs do not always show on the x-ray. If the patient has point tenderness over a rib and the x-ray is negative, there still may be a hairline fracture — treat accordingly.
- Assume that a patient with fractures of ribs 1-3 has a severe underlying injury until proven otherwise.
- If at least five ribs are fractured or if at least three ribs are fractured in two different places, a flail chest is present.
- Bony lesions of the ribs are most likely due to metastatic tumor.

The Abdomen:

Moans and Groans

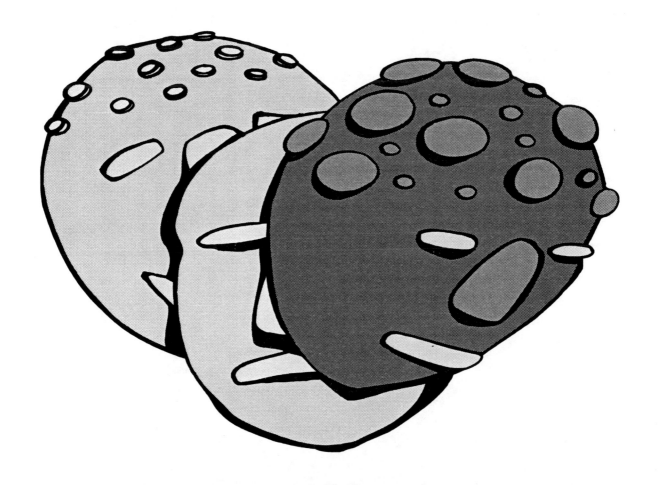

THE ABDOMEN — MOANS AND GROANS

CHAPTER OUTLINE

The Abdomen — Moans and Groans
    The Normal Abdominal Film
    Abnormal Air Shadows
        Free Intraperitoneal "Air"
        Motility Disturbances
    Abnormal Water Shadows
    Funny Looking Things
        Tubes
        Foreign Bodies
        Abnormal Calcifications
        Constipation
    Summary — Rules of the Abdomen

LEARNING OBJECTIVES

After completing this chapter, you'll be able to:

1. Describe the appearance of a normal abdominal x-ray series.

2. Analyze an x-ray and judge if an NG tube is in correct position.

3. In the abdominal x-ray series:

    A. Describe and recognize abnormal gas collections.
    B. Describe and recognize abnormal bowel gas patterns.
    C. Describe and recognize abnormal calcifications.

4. State two common abnormal conditions that are easily seen on the routine abdominal series.

THE NORMAL ABDOMINAL FILM

Abdominal films are *even easier* than most chest x-rays! As in the chest, think of the belly as a tree. The trunk of the tree is the vertebral column, and the base is the upper pelvis. The tree trunk is supported on each side by the

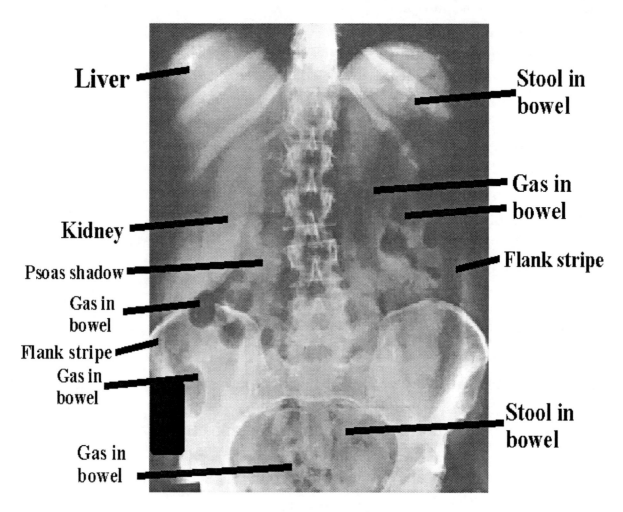

Liver

Stool in bowel

Gas in bowel

Kidney

Flank stripe

Psoas shadow

Gas in bowel

Flank stripe

Gas in bowel

Stool in bowel

Gas in bowel

Figure A-1

psoas muscle shadows while the lower ribs form the upper branches of the tree (Figure A-1). Almost reminds me of a rain forest, with a canopy above and "guts" down below! Our forest is pretty windy,

REMEMBER — The psoas shadows should be relatively distinct. Otherwise, look for overlying stool or intraperitoneal fluid.

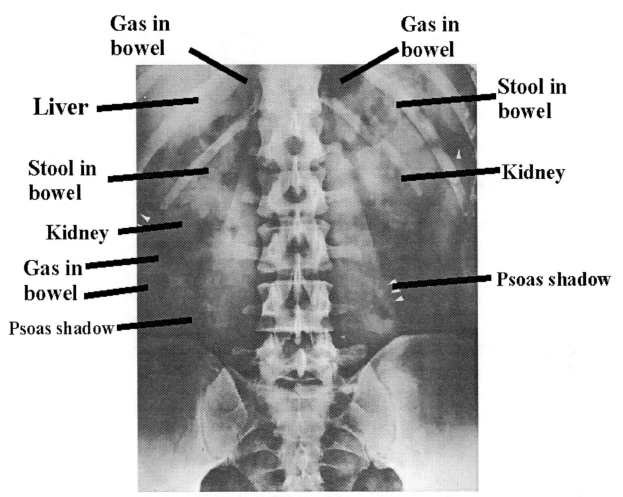

Gas in bowel

Gas in bowel

Liver

Stool in bowel

Stool in bowel

Kidney

Kidney

Gas in bowel

Psoas shadow

Psoas shadow

Figure A-2

so think of the psoas shadows as supports for the "vertebral tree." Normally, these should be fairly clear. Sometimes, though, stool obliterates part of them. If there is no obvious stool and the psoas shadows are *still* fuzzy or invisible, the most likely cause is intraperitoneal fluid (Figure A-2).

The most interesting thing about the normal abdominal film is that you don't see a lot of what? Bowel — gas-filled bowel, which looks like balloons, is conspicuously *absent*. You may see a few loops of large bowel, but

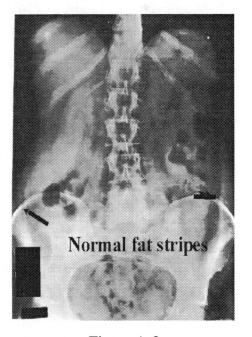

Normal fat stripes

Figure A-3

lots of dark shadows in the belly are abnormal. Remember, dark shadows indicate either gas or fat — despite most of our concerns with "fat stomachs," this kind of fat shadow is *not* seen on the x-ray. So, dark shadows within the abdomen are often gas in the bowel. An exception to this rule is the normal **flank fat stripes** usually seen bilaterally. Sometimes, though not always, obliteration of one of these may be a sign of intraperitoneal fluid. More commonly, though, stool or gas in the large bowel "blurs out" the flank fat stripe (Figure A-3).

> *REMEMBER* — "Balloons" in the belly are usually abnormal!

What you *do* see in the normal belly film are lots of soft tissue shadows. The psoas muscle shadows should be clear along their entire length. Sometimes, the kidney, liver, and spleen shadows are visible. By the way, quite often you see fluffy mid-density material throughout the abdomen. What is it? You guessed — poop! Remember, the passage of stool in various stages of formation is part of our normal bodily functions. Unless a patient was kind enough to take a "bowel prep" before getting sick or injured, the normal abdominal film is bound to have at least *some* stool visible. Don't make the mistake of assuming that just because you see stool, the patient's main diagnosis is constipation. A true x-ray diagnosis of F.O.S. ("full of stool") is difficult to make (see below).

> *REMEMBER* — Just because you see stool in the abdomen doesn't mean the patient has constipation!

ABNORMAL AIR SHADOWS

The most important abnormal air shadows on the abdominal film are also some of the easiest to see — free intraperitoneal "air" (free "air") and motility disturbances.

Free intraperitoneal "air" —
Think about the diaphragm shadows again... remember we're seeing not a single structure, but a conglomeration of diaphragm-liver-spleen-stomach (depending on the side, of course). Normally, we don't see an interface between them because they have the same density. And, at the point where two materials of the *same* radiographic density meet, there is *no* interface ("BILL!").

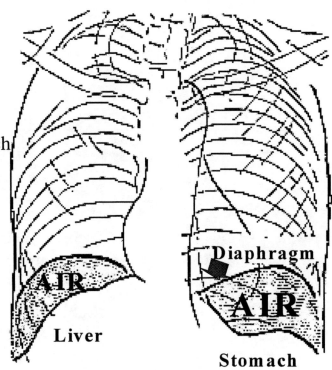

Air "dissects" between the liver or stomach and the diaphragm, causing an interface that outlines the "paper-thin" diaphragm.

Figure A-4

If air is introduced into the peritoneal cavity (**pneumoperitoneum**) and the patient is in an upright position, what happens? Air will "float" upwards and stop beneath the diaphragm. Now, we have diaphragm-air-organs (liver, spleen, stomach). In other words, now there is an *interface* ("BILL") present because air has a different radiodensity than the diaphragm or other organs (Figure A-4). Think about it — when this happens, the diaphragm appears "paper-thin." And, you'll remember one of our earlier rules: "The diaphragm should never be paper-thin; if it is, there's abnormal air within... the peritoneum!" This is why an upright chest x-ray is almost always part of the typical abdominal x-ray series — to look for free air under the diaphragm (Figure A-5).

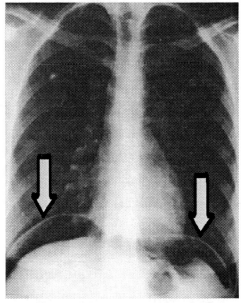

Figure A-5 — "Paper-thin" diaphragm due to free intraperitoneal air.

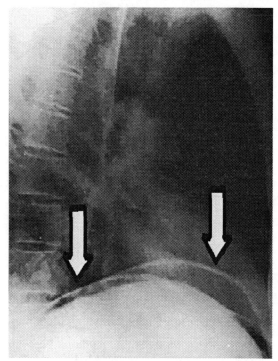

Figure A-6 — Lateral view showing "paper-thin" diaphragm shadows...

Technically speaking, free "air" is a *finding* while "ruptured viscus" represents a *diagnosis*. Other things may also result in free "air" (bowel trauma, post-surgical).

Sometimes small amounts of air are introduced during laparoscopy, open abdominal surgery, gynecological procedures, and even following water skiing in women (air is forced from the vagina into the uterus and tubes, then into the peritoneal cavity after a hard fall). If, however, the patient presents with an acute abdominal complaint and you see a paper-thin diaphragm— guess what? He or she has intraperitoneal free "air" (gas) due to rupture of a hollow viscus until proven otherwise. Often, though not always, the perforated viscus is a peptic ulcer. Interestingly, one in six people who present with perforated peptic ulcers have *no* prior ulcer history — perforation *is* their first presentation. Regardless of the cause, when you see a paper thin diaphragm think ruptured or perforated hollow viscus!

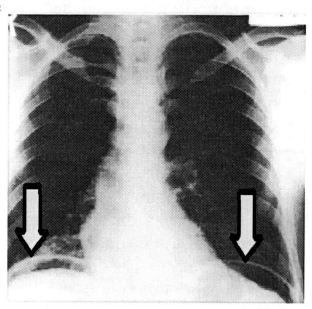

Bilateral "paper-thin" diaphragm indicating intraperitoneal free air...

Figure A-7

Free air may be visible under one or both hemidiaphragms and when present, is a very reliable sign (Figures A-6, A-7). It is only visible in 85% of cases of documented hollow viscus rupture! If you strongly suspect the presence of rupture and don't see free air on the x-ray, try getting a noncontrast abdominal CT scan — very small amounts of intraperitoneal free air are seen as very dark "spots" in the belly. You just can't miss it!

Motility disturbances — Collectively, this term refers to both bowel obstruction and ileus. The term **bowel obstruction** implies a physical blockage while **ileus** suggests a localized or generalized decrease in muscle contraction of the bowel wall due to any of a number of things. I prefer the more generic descriptor because, quite frankly, it's difficult to tell one from the other on many x-rays. And, from a clinical point of view it doesn't matter... at least early on. The clinical treatment for either disorder consists of nothing by mouth (NPO), IV fluids, nasogastric suction, and prompt surgical consultation if the patient's not better in a couple of days.

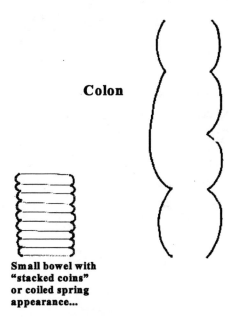

Colon

Small bowel with "stacked coins" or coiled spring appearance...

Figure A-8

Though it's not absolutely essential to differentiate "obstruction" from "ileus" most of the time, sometimes you get a pretty good idea based on the gas pattern:

- If there is localized bowel distension (e.g., small bowel only), suspect mechanical obstruction.

> *REMEMBER* — "Motility disturbance" is a *finding*; "obstruction" or "ileus" is a *diagnosis*...

- If there is a part of the bowel at which distension abruptly stops (such as the mid-transverse colon) *and* the rectum is empty with no gas present, suspect mechanical obstruction.

- If *all* parts of the bowel and the stomach are dilated, suspect ileus.

When a motility disturbance is present, what happens? "Stuff" backs up in the intestines and they dilate, filled with gas and fluid. Depending on the view angle, you see one of two pictures — dilated bowel alone or air-fluid levels (technically speaking, "gas-fluid levels") in dilated loops of bowel. Dilated small bowel has lines visible across the entire width, while large bowel does not (Figure A-8). Typically, you don't see small bowel

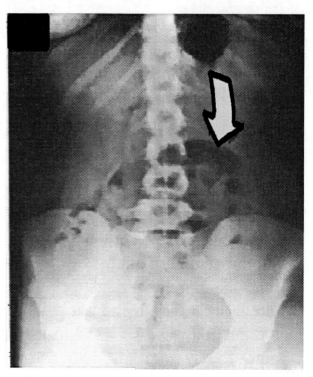

"Bent-finger" sign indicating localized ileus in small bowel...

Figure A-9

on the normal film; if you do, it's limited to one or two small loops that are less than 2.5 cm in width [Murfitt, J., "*The Acute Abdomen*," in: A Short Textbook of Clinical Imaging, Sutton D, and Young, JRW, editors; Springer-Verlag; London 1990; p. 431].

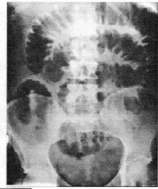
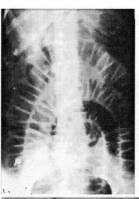
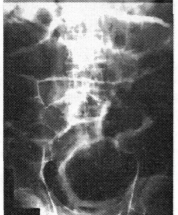
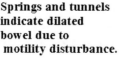

Springs and tunnels indicate dilated bowel due to motility disturbance.

Figure A-10

Even *one* isolated loop of small bowel *may* be abnormal, overlying an irritated viscus, such as the appendix. In this case, it's often referred to as a "sentinel loop," or "bent-finger sign," and represents a localized ileus due to inflammation (Figure A-9).

So, dilated small bowel looks a lot like "springs" and together with dilated large bowel forms a series of layered "tunnels." Thus, the "ST changes" of motility disturbance are ***springs and tunnels*** (Figure A-10). When you see these, you should strongly suspect the presence of a motility disturbance. Look at the film on the right (Figure A-11) — what do you see? Springs and tunnels! Sure hope you're considering a motility disturbance when you see this picture.

In other views, trapped fluid in dilated loops of bowel may be visible as air-fluid levels. These look somewhat like turtle shells (Figure A-12). So, in this view, the sign of motility disturbance is

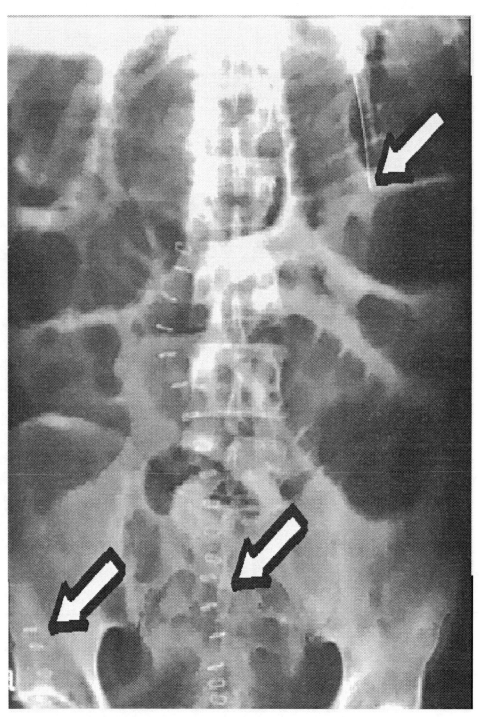

Figure A-11

"turtles"! Taken together, the signs of motility disturbance, then, are springs, tunnels, and turtles. If you remember this, silly as it may sound, you won't miss motility disturbances on an abdominal film.

BY THE WAY — Did you notice the NG tube and surgical staples on the last film (white arrows)??

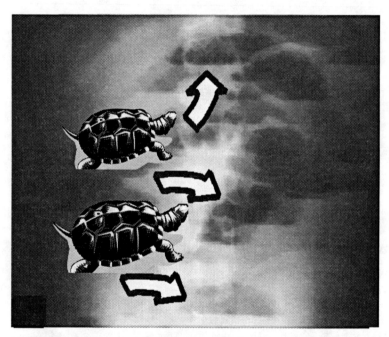

Note the close resemblance of air-fluid levels to the side view of a turtle's shell!

Figure A-12

REMEMBER — The signs of motility disturbance are springs, tunnels, and turtles!

ABNORMAL WATER SHADOWS

If you remember the basic principles we discussed earlier regarding *why* things look the way they do on a film, this one is really easy! Think about it — the normal film has several easily discernable shadows (e.g., psoas muscle). If we put a hose into the abdomen and "fill 'er up," what happens? The fluid co-mingles with the peritoneal contents, all of which have fluid-density. Thus, the normal shadows are all obliterated. Make sense? Good!

Diffuse ascites will blur out all the normal intra-abdominal shadows, resulting in a diffuse hazy appearance of the abdomen (Figure A-13). The amount of fluid varies widely from patient to patient. In fact, fluid in the peritoneal cavity *from any cause* will have the same effect. For example, intra-abdominal bleeding or abscess formation often leads to cloudiness about the affected area. Once you realize that the normal fluid-density shadows have been obliterated, it's easy to surmise that the only substance that could have done that *must also* have

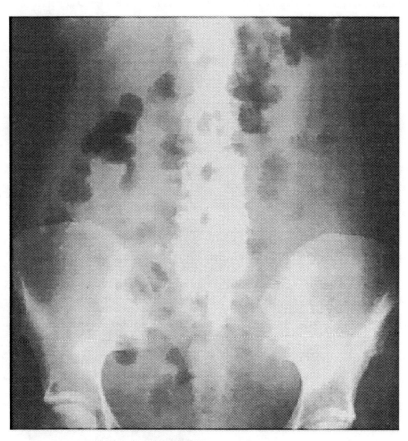

Diffuse abdominal haziness with obliteration of psoas shadows due to intraperitoneal fluid collection.

Figure A-13

fluid-density. Then look at the clinical picture and formulate a differential diagnosis!

FUNNY LOOKING THINGS

Tubes — Nasogastric tubes often contain a radiopaque line to aid in seeing them on x-ray. The tip and side hole should lie beyond the esophagogastric junction and into the stomach (Figures A-14, A-15).

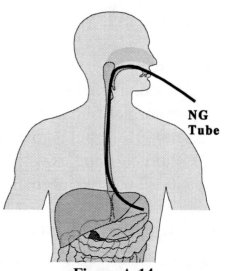

Figure A-14

Foreign bodies — There are numerous potential foreign bodies you may see in any part of the gastrointestinal tract, from the esophagus to the rectum. Particularly in small children, larger swallowed foreign bodies tend to stick in the upper esophagus. They have a characteristic appearance in the PA or AP film. When you see a radiopaque object at the level of the clavicles that appears flat, strongly suspect that it is in the esophagus. This area is the narrowest portion of the entire GI tract and the commonest place for something to "stick."

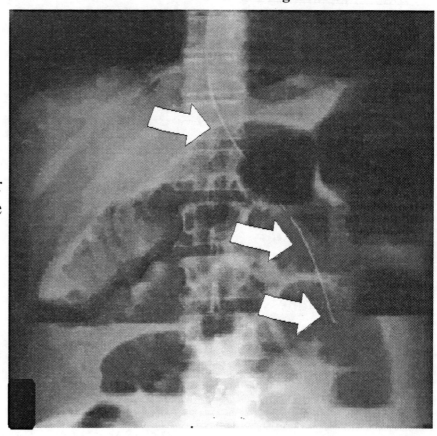

Normally positioned nasogastric tube...

Figure A-15

It's easy to differentiate an esophageal foreign body from one in the trachea. If the object is in the trachea it appears in a plane ninety degrees to that of an impacted esophageal foreign body. The reason? The cartilage rings of the

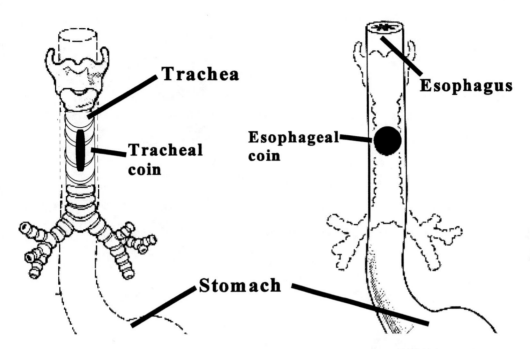

Figure A-16

trachea prevent all but the smallest objects from lying in the same plane as those trapped in the esophagus (Figures A-16, A-17). By the way, most patients with tracheal foreign bodies are rather busy coughing as well!

Abnormal calcifications — Any of a number of conditions can cause abnormal calcifications on the plain abdominal film.

- Chronic pancreatitis forms calcific scars in the islets, leading to a diffuse,

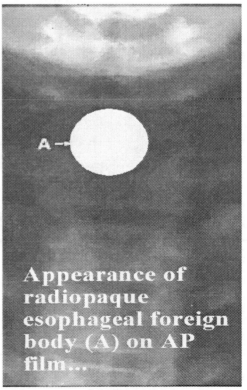

Appearance of radiopaque esophageal foreign body (A) on AP film...

Figure A-17

stippled appearance of the pancreas. You can almost imagine the calcified islet cells (Figure A-18).

- Gallstones are often radiopaque and appear as circular densities in the right upper quadrant of the abdomen, below the ribs (Figure A-19).

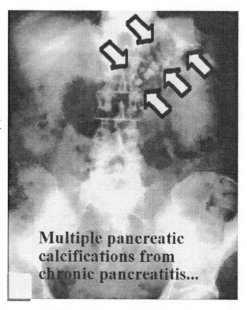

Multiple pancreatic calcifications from chronic pancreatitis...

Figure A-18

- An appendicolith is a piece of feces stuck in the lumen of the appendix. Though this blockage is the cause of appendicitis, seeing an appendicolith on x-ray is uncommon — it's radiopaque and visible in less than ten percent of patients. Now, that's the bad news; the good news is that if you do see an appendicolith in the right lower quadrant and the clinical picture fits, the chances of the surgeon's finding appendicitis are greater than ninety percent!

- Potentially, the most deadly of the list is an abdominal aortic aneurysm (AAA). Though the abdominal x-ray is no longer considered the first-line diagnostic study, eggshell density (usually due to atherosclerotic calcification) in the vicinity of the aorta may present you with the first hint (Figure A-20). If you see this, consider either an ultrasound or abdominal CT scan. If the patient is already leaking enough blood to develop shock,

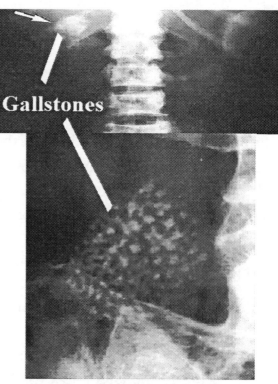

Gallstones

Figure A-19

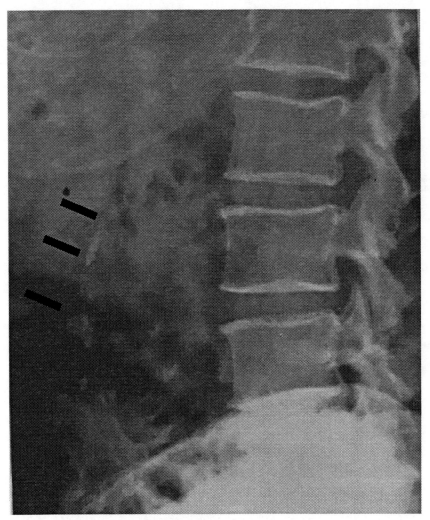

Calcification in anterior aorta suggests AAA!
Figure A-20

rapid operation, not lots of diagnostic studies, offers the best chance to save a life.

Constipation — As I said earlier, it's normal to see at least some stool in the belly film. This does *not* indicate a diagnosis of constipation. Health care providers tend to jump to conclusions without sufficient data. For example, assume we have a patient with belly pain and we've ruled out the possibility of an acute surgical emergency. Now, since the "powers that be" need a diagnosis, what do we usually do? If the patient has nausea, vomiting, *and* diarrhea we call it "gastroenteritis" or "flu." If there isn't any diarrhea, the next step is usually to get a belly film (or look again at the one we got earlier). Chances are excellent that we will see at least a little bit of stool somewhere if we look hard enough. *Voilá* — once we see stool, we immediately jump to the "diagnosis" of what? Constipation. I know it sounds silly, but in over 20 years of practice, I have seen this happen many times. Every now and then, you *can* see a huge fecaloma on x-ray — then, if the clinical picture is compatible, you might be justified in making a diagnosis of you know what...

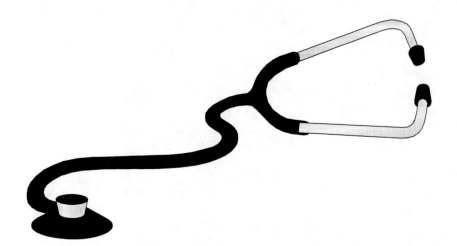

Sounds fishy to me!

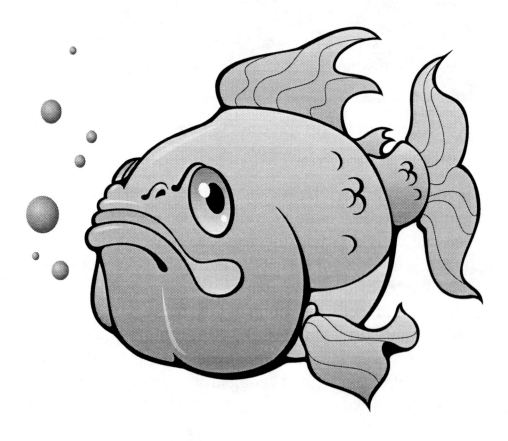

ABD-16

SUMMARY — RULES OF THE ABDOMEN

- In the normal abdominal film, soft tissue shadows and stool are common; gas-filled bowel is not.

- A paper-thin diaphragm shadow on the upright chest film indicates intraperitoneal free air due to ruptured gut until proven otherwise.

- Signs of motility disturbance are springs, tunnels, and turtles.

- Abnormal collections of fluid in the peritoneal cavity obliterate normal soft tissue shadows.

- Eggshell calcification in the vicinity of the aorta is due to abdominal aortic aneurysm until proven otherwise.

- Despite the frequent presence of stool on the abdominal film, don't make the diagnosis of constipation as a "catch-all" diagnosis.

Section 3:

Mostly Bony Injuries

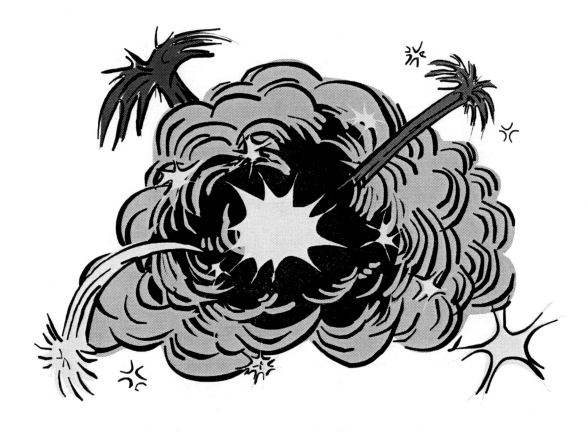

THE BONES — SNAPPY BUT SIMPLE

OUTLINE

The Bones — Snappy but Simple
    Bony Basics — A Review
    Skull and Face
        Skull
        Facial Bones
    The Spine
        Cervical Spine
        Thoracic Spine
        Lumbar Spine
        Sacrum and Coccyx
    The Upper Extremity
        Hand and Wrist
        Forearm
        Elbow
        Arm (Humerus)
        Shoulder, Clavicle, and AC Joint
    The Pelvis and Hips
        Pelvis
        Hips
    The Lower Extremity
        Thigh (Femur)
        Knee
        Leg
        Ankle and Foot
    Summary — Bone Rules!

LEARNING OBJECTIVES

After completing this chapter, you'll be able to:

1.   Recognize the normal lateral skull x-ray.

2.   Differentiate between a skull fracture, a suture, and a vascular marking on the lateral skull film.

3.   Identify x-ray findings of the following conditions: sinusitis, nondepressed skull fracture, depressed skull fracture, fractured mandible, and blow-out fracture of the orbit.

4.   Recognize the appearance of a normal lateral cervical, thoracic, lumbar, sacral, and coccygeal spine x-ray.

5.   Differentiate radiologically stable from radiologically unstable cervical fractures.

6.   Recognize and describe a vertebral compression fracture.

7.   Identify normal x-rays of the following structures: hand, wrist, elbow, arm, shoulder, pelvis, hips, legs, knees, ankle, and foot.

8.   Describe and recognize common fractures and dislocations of the following structures: hand, wrist, elbow, arm, shoulder, pelvis, hips, legs, knees, ankle, and foot.

BONY BASICS — A REVIEW

The principles of making sense of bone x-rays are straightforward. The primary rule is "Bones are smooth; when they're not smooth, they're broken."

So, if you follow the bony

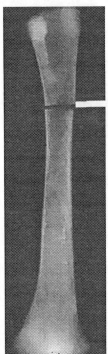

Fracture line...

Figure B-1

> **REMEMBER** — Bones are smooth; when they're not, they're broken!

cortex all the way around any bony shadow, it should be smooth. Suspect a fracture if there are any breaks in the cortex.

The basis for the x-ray appearance of through and through (cortex to cortex) fractures is simple... blood and fat fills in between the distracted fragments (Figure B-1). When an x-ray beam hits, much is attenuated by the radiopaque bone, while the blood-fat mix allows more of the beam through to hit the film. The result — the fracture line appears dark. In addition, since the bony cortex is broken, the bone is no longer smooth.

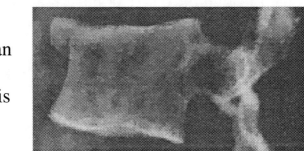

Vertebral compression fracture...

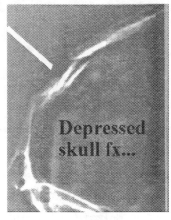

Figure B-2

Other types of fractures involve related principles:

- When bony fragments are impacted or compacted together (e.g., compression fracture, impacted hip fracture), bony density increases. There is more resistance to the passage of x-rays, and a "white line" at the point of bony overlap (Figure B-2).

- In a depressed fracture, the fragment gets in the path of the beam, adding a new opacity (Figure B-2).

- In a **greenstick fracture**, the fracture does *not* extend through the entire bone. There is only a break in one side of the cortex. Sometimes the other side of the bone is buckled together, increasing the bony density, resulting in a denser (whiter) appearance on the x-ray. "Buckling fractures" are also referred to as **torus fractures** (Figure B-3).

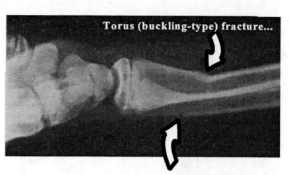

Torus (buckling-type) fracture...

"Greenstick" (not involving the entire bony cortex) fracture...

Figure B-3

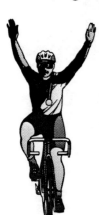

SKULL AND FACE

Both skull and facial bone series tend to be of limited clinical utility, but for

---

Fracture Rules:

- **Are the bones smooth (breaks in the continuity of the cortex)?**

- **Are there radiolucent fracture lines (blood and fat in between the distracted bony fragments)?**

- **Are there abnormally white areas (overlap of cortical and trabecular bone "crushed" together)?**

- **Are there unexplained bony chips (fragments), even if a fracture isn't visible?**

- **Are there dense areas due to impaction of bone?**

different reasons. *None* of us "have a brain" on the normal skull film. In other words, we see a lot of bone but the brain is typically invisible unless there is some unusual mass lesion or calcification present. This fact has led to incorrect diagnostic impressions, especially in children. A normal skull film *does not* rule out intracranial injury (Figure B-4). To do this requires a combination of clinical

REMEMBER — **A normal skull film does not rule out intracranial injury!**

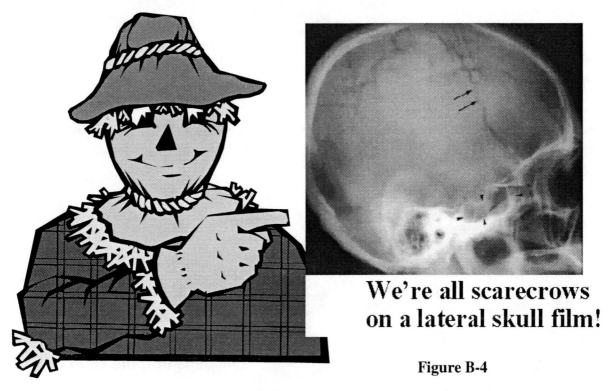

We're all scarecrows on a lateral skull film!

Figure B-4

observation, examination of the patient, and possibly a CT scan. Facial bone x-rays, on the other hand, are just darn hard to make sense out of, even when shot with the most perfect technique.

Skull — The lateral skull x-ray is the most helpful, although an AP view will help to localize abnormal shadows, such as a depressed fracture. There are a couple of

REMEMBER — **"V-fib of the skull" is almost always a normal suture line...**

features of the normal lateral film that may initially be confusing — vascular markings and suture lines. Suture lines form a unique saw-tooth pattern resembling ventricular fibrillation. Thus, "v-fib of the skull" is almost always a suture line.

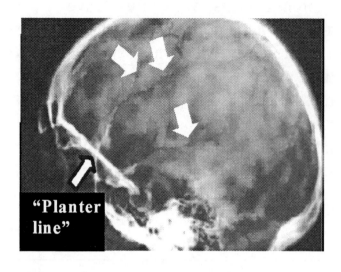

Figure B-5

To appreciate normal vascular markings, draw a line along the base of the skull as shown Figure B-5. Normally, skull vessel markings flow out from this line. Think of it as a garden ("the planter line") and the vessels as plants growing up from it (Figure B-6). The vessels should get smaller as they travel more peripherally, and should all be the same "color." If a line is seen that travels in any other direction, with the exception of a known suture, it's probably a fracture. Similarly, if you see a line that is significantly darker than the rest, suspect a fracture.

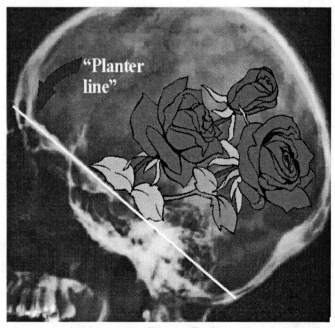

Figure B-6

The skull vessels are embedded in depressed grooves on the inner skull surface. These channels thin the skull, reducing its density. Blood offers less resistance to x-rays than bone, more gets through at the site of the vessels, and more hits the film. The effect — vascular markings appear *darker* than bone. When a fracture is present, there is a "void" through and through the bone, allowing even more x-rays to pass, hitting the film plate, and creating a dark shadow distinctly different from the vessel markings. Finally, if the exposure is such that only a dark line is seen, it is probably a fracture — why? Because the film is likely a bit underexposed, causing the vessels to be relatively invisible. Only the fracture line is seen (Figure B-7). The table below summarizes some important points to help differentiate vascular markings from linear skull fractures.

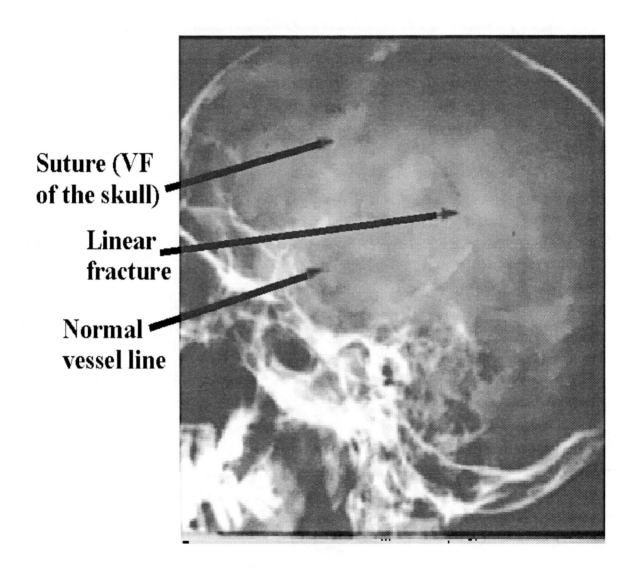

Suture (VF of the skull)

Linear fracture

Normal vessel line

Figure B-7

FRACTURE	VESSEL MARKING
Often appears black due to involvement of both inner and outer tables of bone.	Appears grey because only the inner table of bone is thinned (contains the blood vessels).
Branches don't taper uniformly.	Branches decrease in size peripherally (as they move away from the "planter line").
White (sclerotic) margin absent.	Sclerotic (white) margin usually present.

A skull fracture may be linear, resulting in a radiolucent line as described above, or depressed. Depressed skull fractures occur when a piece of bone pushes into the skull cavity. It may or may not strike the brain. Lateral and AP skull films help you see the fracture. A CT scan verifies the degree of depression and potential brain damage. Masses and foreign bodies appear as easily visible abnormal radiopaque shadows.

Facial bones — The usual "facial series" is often nearly impossible to make any sense out of, except to the most experienced radiologists. Even then, they often recommend supplemental films or additional studies. Many radiographers try and "pin down" the clinician to determine what bone or bones are *really* of interest. Specific shots of specific bones are much more precise than just a "facial bones" series. I'm not going to go into all of the different bones, but will point out two interesting areas, orbital fractures and jaw fractures.

Orbital blow-out fractures occur when a blunt force, such as a baseball or fist, is directed at the globe. The inferior and medial

> *REMEMBER* — Suspect an orbital blow-out fracture with a history of trauma and clouding or air-fluid levels in the maxillary sinus.

walls of the orbit are very thin. To divert trauma from the eye, these bones dissipate the force by fracturing (Figure B-8). Fragments and associated tissue are forced into the underlying maxillary sinus. Hence, the term "blow out"

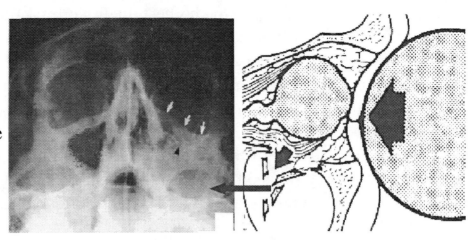

Orbital blow-out fracture leads to clouding of left maxillary sinus...

Figure B-8

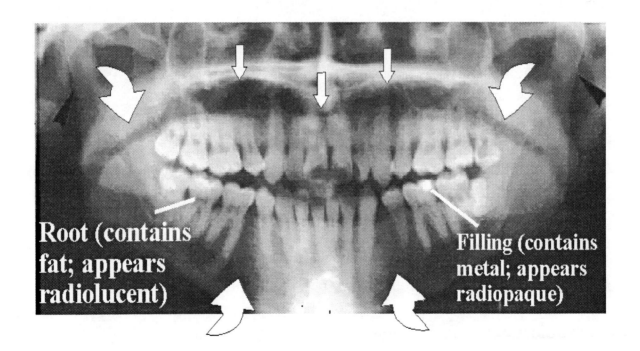

Root (contains fat; appears radiolucent)

Filling (contains metal; appears radiopaque)

Normal Panorex®; arrows point to normal air lines...

Figure B-9

BONES-9

fracture of the orbit. Despite the highest quality orbital films, seeing the fracture line itself is often difficult. On the other hand, indirect signs of the fracture are common. Think about it — if bone and blood collect in the maxillary sinus, what *must* happen? Of course — the sinus appears cloudy or contains an air fluid level on the skull film.

If a patient has a history of trauma, a compatible clinical examination, and an abnormal maxillary sinus on the affected side, assume a blow-out fracture. Clinically, these fractures can trap the inferior oblique muscle or tendon causing paralysis of upward gaze.

Maxillary fractures (Le Fort I, II, and III) are rare and extremely difficult to see without special films (Figure B-10). Clinical acumen is most helpful, since the more serious types (II, III) involve abnormal occlusion of the upper teeth.

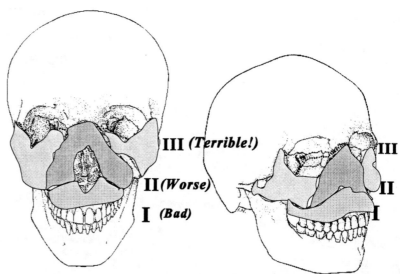

LeFort classification of facial fractures (hard to see on plain films)

Figure B-10

Mandible fractures are best seen on the panoramic-view dental film (Panorex®). Otherwise, the routine mandible view is often difficult to interpret (Figure B-9). Regardless of which film you have access to, the mandible is symmetrical. Follow the cortex of the bones looking for breaks, and fractures should be easy to see. Laterally there are often air shadows which mimic fractures. Check for symmetry — if the shadows are symmetrical *and* the cortices appear smooth, you're probably looking at a normal shadow rather than a fracture.

THE SPINE

Taking the normal curve of the spine into account, you should be able to draw a smooth line along the front and back of the vertebral bodies from the cervical to the lumbar vertebrae. Regardless of which part of the spine you are looking at, the vertebral bodies should always line up along these curved lines (Figures B-11, B-12, B-13). So, the first rule of the spine is "we line up." Use these lines to determine quickly whether proper alignment of the spine is present. Regardless of the portion of the spine in question, if

the front and back of the vertebral bodies don't line up, assume the patient has an **unstable spine** — there is a risk of injury to the spinal cord.

The Vertebral Column, Its Sections and Curves

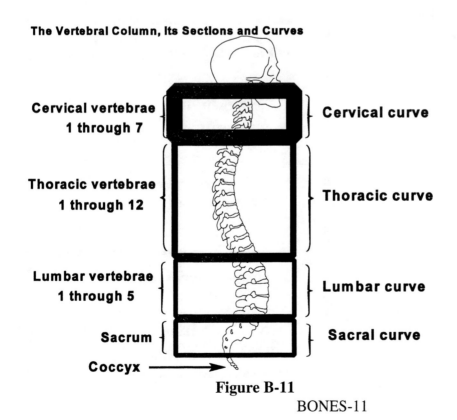

Cervical vertebrae 1 through 7 — Cervical curve

Thoracic vertebrae 1 through 12 — Thoracic curve

Lumbar vertebrae 1 through 5 — Lumbar curve

Sacrum — Sacral curve

Coccyx ⟶

Figure B-11

In addition, the "color" or density of the vertebral bodies should be uniform throughout the vertebral column. Diffuse changes in "color," either too dark or too light, are likely due to systemic metabolic bone disease (such as rickets or osteoporosis). If it is diffusely darkened (increased radiolucency to the entire spine), suspect **osteoporosis**. Isolated changes in the "color" of the vertebral bodies may indicate infection, fracture, tumor, or other injury.

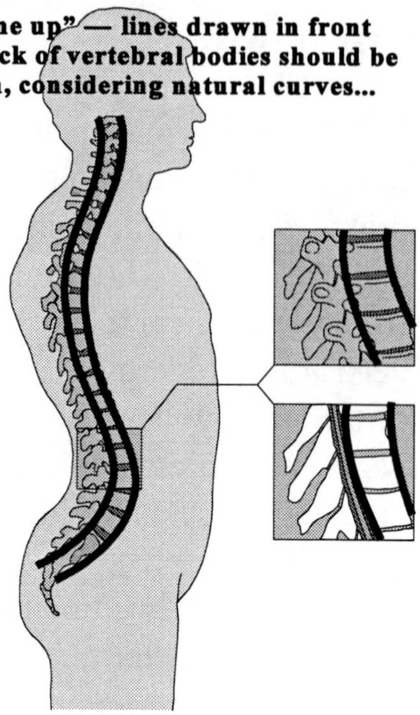

The front height and back height of the vertebral bodies should be just about the same. An exception to this rule sometimes occurs in the thoracic spine where the posterior height may normally be 1-2 mm greater than the anterior height. If so, the finding occurs in *all or most* of the thoracic vertebrae. Isolated differences are *not* normal and are often due, as in other parts of the spine, to a compression fracture.

Figure B-12

With a compression fracture, the anterior height is decreased because the normally square body is wedged into a trapezoid shape.

Another easy way some people use to remember how to see everything in the spine film is the acronym "ABC'S":

- A = **A**lignment and anatomy (do we line up?)

- B = **B**ony integrity (are the bones smooth?)

- C = **C**artilage (is the joint space narrowed?)

- S = **S**oft tissues (is there soft tissue swelling?)

ABC's of Spine Films:

- A = **A**lignment and anatomy (do we line up?)

- B = **B**ony integrity (are the bones smooth?)

- C = **C**artilage (is the joint space narrowed?)

- S = **S**oft tissues (is there soft tissue swelling?)

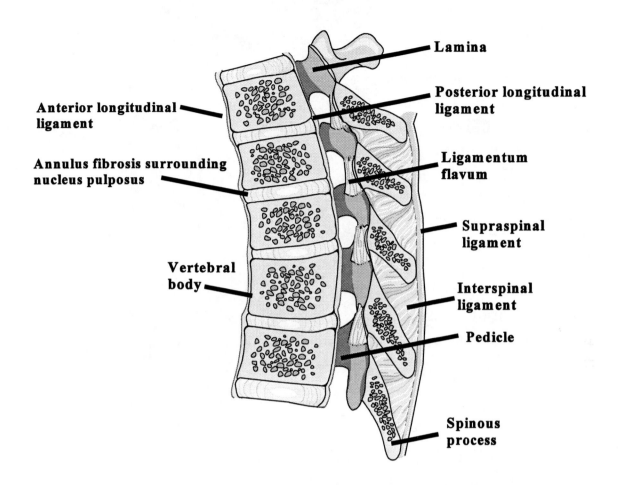

Anterior longitudinal ligament

Annulus fibrosis surrounding nucleus pulposus

Vertebral body

Lamina

Posterior longitudinal ligament

Ligamentum flavum

Supraspinal ligament

Interspinal ligament

Pedicle

Spinous process

Figure B-13

The spine is a common location for **degenerative osteoarthritis**. This causes formation of excess bone, particularly on the anterior portions of the vertebral bodies. These **arthritic spurs** or **osteophytes** are essentially "scar bone" formed by excess stress on the intervertebral joints, and inflammation. The interspaces contain the intervertebral disks, though the disks themselves are *not* visible on plain films (Figure B-14). Disc degeneration or injury, though, may lead to narrowing of one or more interspaces. In the lumbar spine, the interspaces normally widen slightly from L1-L2 to L4-L5. Narrowing of the interspace is the most common x-ray finding correlated with symptomatic lower back pain.

The most frequently injured area is the lumbosacral spine, followed by the cervical spine. The thoracic spine is rarely injured with the exception of relatively minor compression fractures. The reason is that the surrounding ribs and intrathoracic muscles "splint" the spine and prevent excessive movements. Severe disruptions of the thoracic spine require massive trauma.

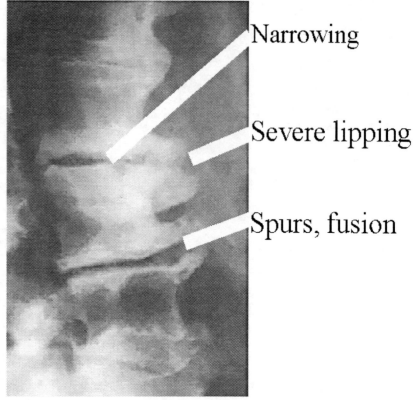

Narrowing

Severe lipping

Spurs, fusion

Figure B-14

Cervical spine — Of course, the major concern with cervical spine (C-spine) injuries is spinal cord damage. Remember, the cord runs in the spinal canal posterior to the vertebral body and is bordered on either side by the lamina. There are several muscles and ligaments between each vertebra. Damage to any of these may result in spinal instability and subluxation (slippage) of a portion of the C-spine over another. Though you should always check for bony damage as well (are the bones smooth?), disruption of the ligaments *alone* can lead to cord-threatening injuries. Remember, the vertebral bodies should "line up." In addition to the two lines in front and in back of the vertebral body we've already talked about, there's one additional line you can use on the C-spine (Figures B-15, B-16). The three lines are:

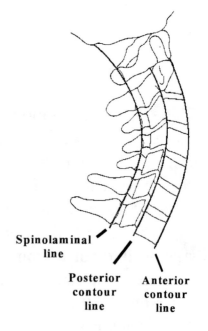

Spinolaminal line

Posterior contour line

Anterior contour line

Figure B-15

- A line drawn along the anterior margins of the cervical vertebral bodies (**anterior contour line**).

- A line drawn along the posterior margins of the cervical vertebral bodies; this line outlines the anterior margin of the spinal canal (**posterior contour line**).

- A line drawn along the anterior margins of the bases of the spinous processes; this line outlines the posterior margin of the spinal canal and is sometimes called the **spinolaminal line.**

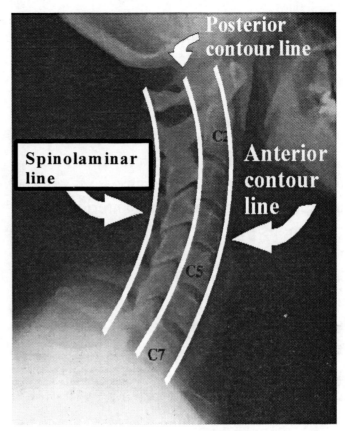

The three normal lines of contour in the C-spine...

Figure B-16

The beauty of these lines is two-fold. First of all, it's a snap (no pun intended) to determine quickly whether "we line up" or not. If the bones don't line up, the patient has an unstable spine — period! Second, the lines automatically draw your eyes across the entire vertebra and related structures, from anterior to posterior. They force you to look at everything — you won't miss, say, an isolated spinous process fracture.

Before checking alignment, remember the "IQAWBF" acronym — the *quality* of a lateral neck film is best when you are easily able to see *all* seven cervical vertebrae, as well as at least part of T-1 (Figure B-17). Otherwise, you are likely to miss something. There are various tricks that radiographers can do to help see C7 in a difficult patient — work together as colleagues to find a solution (Figure B-18).

Once you've checked alignment, verify whether the bony margins are smooth or not. In the cervical spine, any disruption of bony integrity anterior to the spinous processes, whether the bodies line up or not, is to be considered potentially unstable. These rules vary slightly for different parts of the spine (see below).

Even *if* the vertebral bodies line up, and the bones *are* smooth, there are a couple of additional signs that suggest significant bony damage in the cervical spine film:

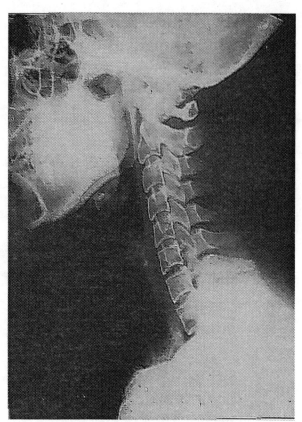

Figure B-17 — Normal Lateral Neck

- Soft tissue swelling — the **prevertebral space** is the x-ray shadows anterior to the vertebral bodies; from C1 - C4 should be no wider than 7 mm or one-third the width of the vertebral body; below the larynx, from C5 - C7, the normal space is wider — no greater than 21 mm or 100% of the width of the vertebral body (Figure B-19). Even if a fracture or misalignment is not seen, widening of this space in a trauma patient is likely due to soft tissue bleeding secondary to an occult cervical spine fracture. Of interest, patients with

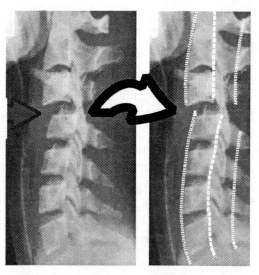

We DON'T line up!

Figure B-18

nontraumatic neck problems, such as retropharyngeal abscess, may also demonstrate prevertebral swelling, though for a very different reason (Figure B-20).

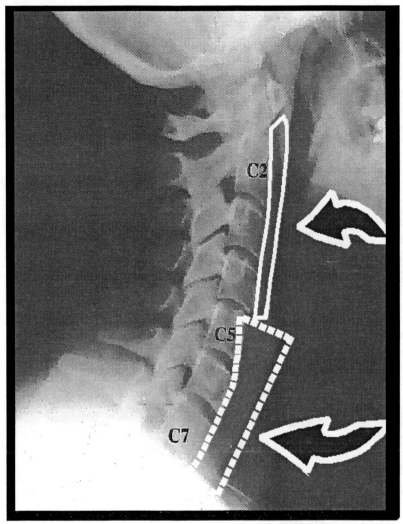

Normal prevertebral soft tissue space widths

C1-C4 — < 7 mm or 1/3 vertebral body width

C5-C7 — < 21 mm or 100% vertebral body width

Figure B-19

- Loose bodies — though true in any joint, if you see small chips or fragments of bone in the interspaces, or anterior to/posterior to the vertebral bodies, the most likely explanation is an occult fracture.

- Straightening or reversal of the normal curve — this principle applies to all parts of the spine (Figure B-21). Remember, the rule "we line up" is based also on the normal curvature. Even if the bodies line up *and* the bones are smooth, straightening or reversal of any part of the normal spinal curves is often due to muscle spasm. Combined with clinical findings, this may indicate an occult fracture. Unfortunately, this finding is not as reliable as the others, because many persons without spinal injury will demonstrate some straightening or even reversal of the curve, particularly in the neck, following immobilization on a spine board.

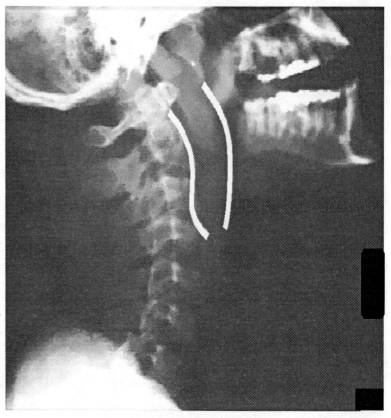

Prevertebral soft tissue swelling C1-C4 (bones smooth)

Figure B-20

Some books use various eponyms (people's names) to describe neck fractures — I have deliberately avoided these terms here because they're easy to forget and to confuse. It's better to describe disruption of the bony ring of C1,

REMEMBER — Be sure you see all seven cervical vertebrae, as well as T-1, before trying to reach any conclusions about the lateral neck film...

than just say "Jefferson fracture" (or is it the Lincoln fracture???). The same principle holds for fractures involving other parts of the body (what is the name of the doggie fracture in the wrist anyway???).

Another issue that comes up all the time is "when should I get a lateral C-spine film?" The typical scenario is a patient who is brought into the Emergency Department in full spinal immobilization after a fall or crash. The yield on routine lateral neck films in this patient population is fairly low — of course, the risk of missing a spinal injury is also great in some cases. The good news is that several studies

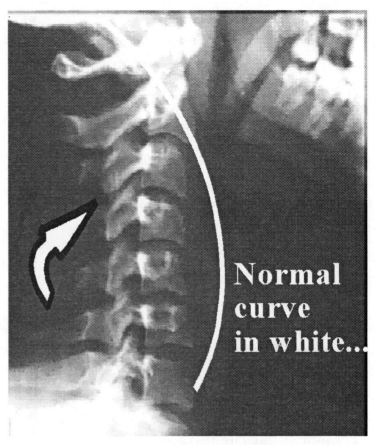

Reversal of the normal cervical curve — no fx seen; film ABNORMAL!!

Figure B-21

Subtle Signs of C-Spine Fractures:

- **Soft tissue swelling in the prevertebral space.**

- **Loose bodies.**

- **Straightening or reversal of the normal curve.**

have provided guidelines as to when a patient *does not* require a film and may be safely removed from spinal immobilization.

Blunt trauma patients may not require cervical spine x-rays if they meet the following criteria: absence of mental status changes, intoxication, neck pain or tenderness, neurologic signs or symptoms, or simultaneous major distracting injury [Foley, K., et.al., Roentgenographic evaluation of the cervical spine. A selective approach; Arch Surg 1994 Jun;129(6):643-5]. Please remember that these criteria are *not* accepted in all areas and by all clinicians!

Look at the figure below (Figure B-22A); after convincing yourself that, indeed, seven cervical vertebrae are visible, check for alignment. What do you think? The report said "normal." Do you agree? Seems to me that there is some malalignment

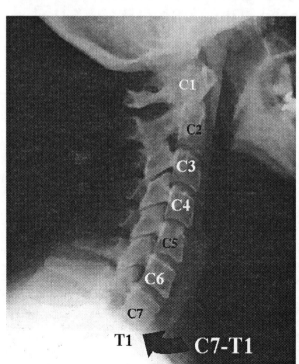

Figure B-22A

Approach to the C-Spine Film

- **Do I see all seven cervical vertebrae and part of T-1?**

- **Do we line up? (Is there straightening or reversal of the normal curve?)**

- **Are the bones smooth? (Are loose bodies present?)**

- **Are the front and back heights of the vertebral bodies equal?**

- **Is there prevertebral space swelling?**

posteriorly at the C3-C4 junction. In addition, the anterior line looks "funny" in front of C4 and C5. There is prevertebral space swelling anterior to C5 and C6. Now, are the bones smooth? Looks like it. This is an *abnormal* film, despite the incorrect reading on the "chart." The lack of normal bony alignment and the prevertebral swelling suggest an occult fracture if this patient suffered neck trauma (see Figure B-22B for an annotated version of this film).

The lateral film will show up to 95% of major pathology of the neck, if present. Of course, a complete series includes more films. The x-ray views routinely obtained differ from department to department. Always make certain that you have ample views to see what you need to see. If you do not, ask the radiographer for suggestions.

Thoracic spine — The most helpful view of the thoracic spine (T-spine) is the lateral. In fact, this view is the *one* best view for all areas of the vertebral column. Use the two lines anterior and posterior to the vertebral bodies, as for the C-spine, to

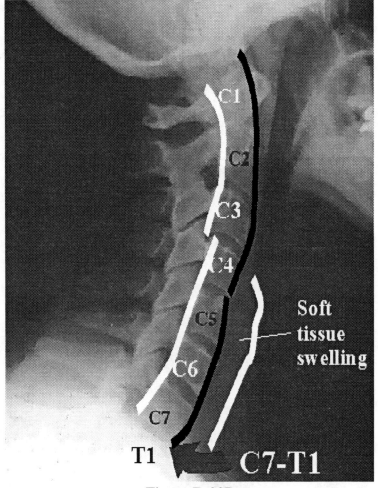

Figure B-22B

verify that accounting for the normal curve, the vertebral bodies line up. As I mentioned earlier, you should make a habit of using lines in *all* areas of the

spine to make certain that "we line up." Remember always to follow each vertebra posteriorly all the way to the end of the spinous process. Make the front to back scan a habit in *every* area of the spine you look at.

> *REMEMBER* — The anterior height of the thoracic vertebral bodies may be slightly (1-2 mm) less than the posterior height in the lateral view; this is normal, as long as the majority of the 12 vertebrae show the same difference...

The only major difference in the thoracic spine is that sometimes, as noted earlier, the posterior body height is normally slightly higher than the anterior height. So, don't automatically jump to the conclusion that there are twelve compression fractures! Only suspect a compression fracture if the

REMEMBER — **Always scan from front to back, covering the entire spine, regardless of which part you are viewing...**

disparity in anterior versus posterior height is different than the rest. Also look for other signs of compression fractures (Figure B-23). The rib shadows overlap those of the vertebrae, and may cause confusion. In your mind, follow the cortices of the ribs as they overlap the vertebral bodies to determine whether you are just seeing overlapping shadows or if an

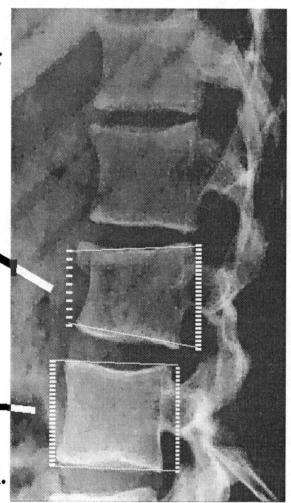

Normal vs Compression Fx

Vertebral compression fracture; anterior (front) height less than posterior (back) height; shaped like a trapezoid.

Normal square to rectangular-shaped vertebral body; front and back heights equal.

Figure B-23

BONES-22

abnormality is present. Compression fractures occur as a result of hyperflexion of the spine and are the most common bony injury to the thoracic vertebrae. Think about what happens — as the spine is flexed forward, forces are directed primarily against the anterior part of the vertebral body. The fracture line usually extends in an anterior-posterior direction causing disruption of both cortices. It may be visible across the entire vertebral body, but most commonly is best seen in the very anterior and very posterior portions.

In addition, the compression forces cause the bone to compact ("crunch") together in the mid-body region. What would you expect on the film? Well, now we have pieces of bone more tightly compacted, which increases their radiographic density. An x-ray beam will find more resistance to passage at this

> ## *Anatomy of a Compression Fracture*
>
> - **Fracture line best seen in very anterior, very posterior portions (the snake's "tail").**
>
> - **Bone "crunches together" centrally forming the "snake's eye."**
>
> - **Mid-body bone pushed centrally, causing "fang bone" of upper anterior body.**

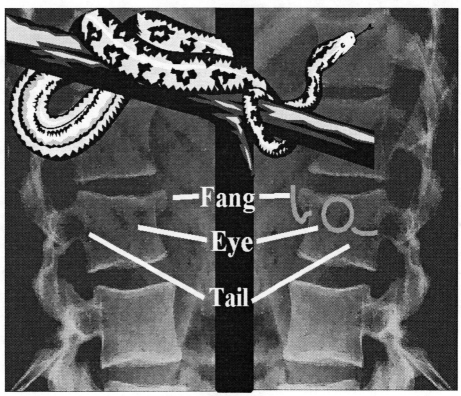

Figure B-24

point, leading to less hitting the film plate. The result? This area is more radiopaque and appears *whiter* on the film! Sometimes, the rib overlies this area, making it difficult to pick out the increased density. The easiest trick is to compare the apparently abnormal vertebra with an obviously normal one. The anterior portion of the fracture is often driven inwards, leaving the

> *REMEMBER* — **Isolated compression fractures rarely cause neurological compromise, unless there is also misalignment of the spine.**

superior part sticking out, much like a reptile's fang (the "fang sign"). Though this "fang" is usually easy to see, you won't miss even a subtle one if you carefully follow the outlines of the bone cortex. Remember — bones are smooth. And when they're not? They're broken! Together, reminds me of a snake (Figure B-24) — the fracture line ("snake's tail"), the central compression ("snake's eye"), and the overlapping anterior bone ("fang").

Lumbar spine — Most injuries to this area of the back involve soft tissues. No surprise that lower back pain is one of the commonest maladies to present to health care providers. It is also a leading cause of workers' compensation and disability claims in the court system. Like the cervical and thoracic spine, the principles of alignment and smooth bones apply in the lumbar spine (L-spine). The interspaces tend to widen from the L1-L2 space to the L4-L5

We STILL line up!

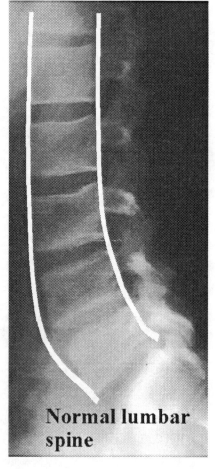

Normal lumbar spine

Figure B-25

space. As you evaluate alignment and bony smoothness, be sure to look at the entire vertebra, anterior to posterior (Figure B-25).

There is much current debate concerning the value of routine lumbosacral (LS) spine x-rays in patients with low back pain. Depending on the study, anywhere from 50 - 85% of persons *without* any symptoms have abnormal LS spine x-rays, most commonly showing degenerative changes. So, it is difficult to determine if the findings were responsible for the patient's pain or not. Many authorities have recommended that unless there is direct trauma, neurologic abnormalities, or you suspect malignancy, then routine L-S spine films are not necessary in the first four weeks for patients with low back pain. [M.W. van Tulder, et.al., Spinal radiographic findings and nonspecific low back pain. A systematic review of observational studies. Spine 22:427-34; (Feb 15, 1997)].

Sacrum and coccyx — Though these areas don't have perceptible vertebral bodies, per se, the rule of alignment still applies. Both sacrum and coccyx should follow a smooth line, again taking into account the body's natural curvature. As before, the bony cortices should be smooth.

THE UPPER EXTREMITITY

The basic rule of bones (bones are smooth...) remains the backbone (no pun intended) of looking at extremity films. In both the upper and lower extremities, the areas of most interest are the joints. The long bones in between are pretty darn simple to make sense out of — either they're smooth or they're not.

Hand — The metacarpals and phalanges are easy — they line up, and the cortices are smooth. Otherwise, they are *often* (though not always!) either dislocated or fractured. The spaces at the interphalangeal (IP) and metacarpal-phalangeal

> *REMEMBER* — **The MCP and IP joints should all be about one millimeter wide...**

(MCP) joints should be uniform and about one mm each (Figure B-26). Narrowing of this space on the AP view may indicate a severe misalignment, only seen on a lateral view. Remember — "one view is one view too few!"

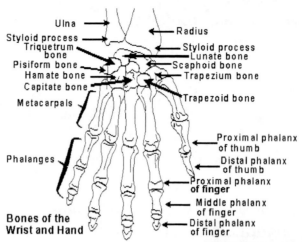

Bones of the Wrist and Hand

Fractures and dislocations of the fingers are fairly easy to see. In fact, they tend to be downright attention-getting. I call injuries like these "major orthopedic turn-ons" (MOTs). The reason? Generally, they get our attention quickly, yet may *not* be the most important finding. Take, for example, the patient with

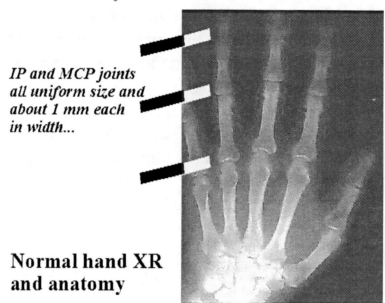

IP and MCP joints all uniform size and about 1 mm each in width...

Normal hand XR and anatomy

Figure B-26

REMEMBER — Our priorities for patient care are always Airway, Breathing, and Circulation!

---

an open wrist fracture — tends to get the whole Emergency Department crew in a nice semicircle to look. Only one problem — that fracture won't, in the absence of other more severe injuries, kill *anyone*. If we get too distracted looking at the MOT, we might just miss the airway obstruction that the patient has as well! The "A" in ABC stands for "Airway," *not* for "Arm." And, you'd be surprised at how often this *still* happens... enough said.

There are three soft tissue structures in the fingers that are at high risk for injury, especially during a dislocation — extensor tendons, volar plates, collateral ligaments (medial and lateral). Each of these attach to the bone, and may be avulsed during trauma. Since they are primarily soft tissues, the avulsed tendon, volar plate, or collateral ligament is *not* visible on x-ray. On the other hand (every pun intended this time), when a soft structure is avulsed away from its point of attachment to the bone, a chip of bone remains attached to the tendon (Figure B-27). And, you *will* be able to see the bony fragment. So, if you see bony fragments, suspect damage to the appropriate extensor tendon, volar

plate, or collateral ligament (Figure B-28). These injuries, though often far less impressive than dislocations or fractures, are *significantly* more important because improper treatment may lead to life-long disability. I strongly suggest you consult a hand surgeon when these injuries are present.

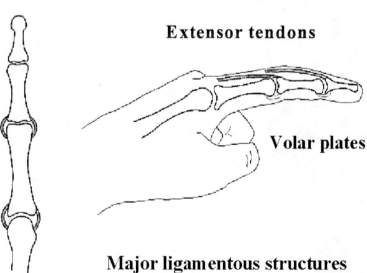

Extensor tendons

Volar plates

Collateral ligaments (medial and lateral)

Major ligamentous structures of the fingers that do *not* show on x-rays; look for avulsion chips!

Figure B-27

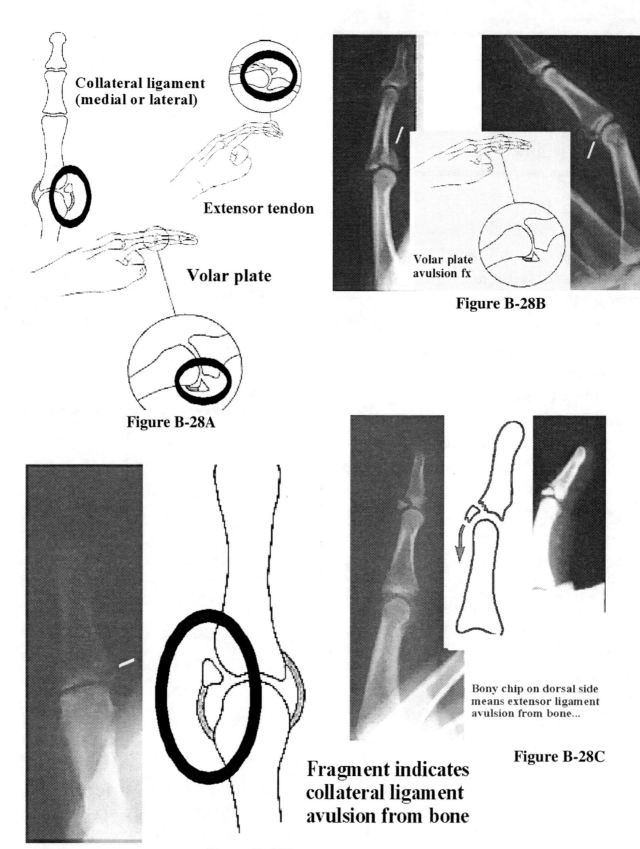

Collateral ligament
(medial or lateral)

Extensor tendon

Volar plate

Figure B-28A

Volar plate
avulsion fx

Figure B-28B

Bony chip on dorsal side
means extensor ligament
avulsion from bone...

Figure B-28C

**Fragment indicates
collateral ligament
avulsion from bone**

Figure B-28D

Often, there is a small round bone seen near the interphalangeal joint of the thumb — sometimes mistaken for a fracture fragment, it's really a **sesamoid bone**. These are located within tendons, and the biggest one in the body is the patella (more on that later). The easiest way to differentiate sesamoid bones from fractures is that sesamoids have nice, smooth borders.

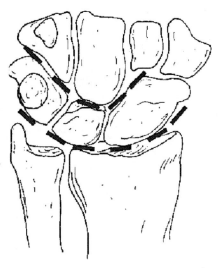 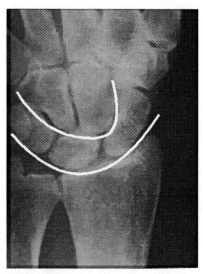

Normal lines of carpal alignment on AP view...

Figure B-29

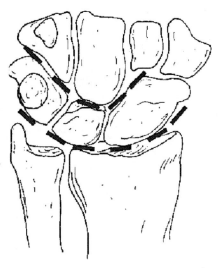

Normal wrist; note normal navicular fat stripe...

Figure B-30

Wrist — On the AP wrist film, the carpal bones should line up. If everything's in the proper alignment, you should be able to draw two "u-shaped" lines below the top and bottom rows (Figures B-29, B-30). In addition, on the lateral wrist film, you should "never see the moon in the wrist." I will explain the significance of this shortly... hang in there!

The most commonly fractured bone in the wrist is the **navicular** or **scaphoid bone** ("N" on normal PA film on the left). It's palpable in the **anatomic snuff box** of the wrist (Figure B-31). Any patient who has a wrist injury and is tender over the navicular bone has a fracture until proven otherwise. And, it's not just as easy as taking a film... navicular fractures tend to be very difficult to see on x-rays, even with special navicular views. Thus, if you suspect a navicular injury, consider immobilizing the thumb and wrist (e.g., thumb spica splint) *regardless* of what the

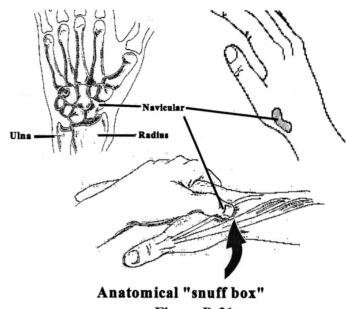

Anatomical "snuff box"
Figure B-31

film shows. The reason? The distal portion of the navicular bone has no independent blood supply. If a fracture is missed, the bone is likely to develop avascular

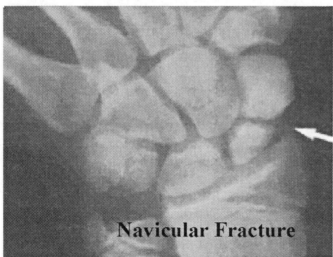

Navicular Fracture

Figure B-32

necrosis. Subsequent disabling osteoarthritis may require a bone transplant and result in severe disability. And, if you're the "lucky one" to miss this fracture, you may also be explaining your reasoning in court. Missed navicular fractures are a *common* cause of litigation involving primary care and emergency care providers. Some fractures of the navicular, however, *are* visible on x-ray. There are no special tricks

— if the bone's not smooth, it's broken (Figure B-32).

Another wrist injury is a carpal bone dislocation. The most commonly dislocated carpal bone is the lunate.

REMEMBER — Assume that any patient with navicular tenderness has a fracture, regardless of the x-ray findings!

There are two primary types of lunate dislocation, lunate and perilunate. Rather than try and remember these, it's easiest to recognize that there is a carpal bone dislocation and get orthopedic assistance. The way to do this is simple, and I've mentioned it earlier — *you should never see the moon in the wrist; if you do, there is a "lunate bone twist"*! By the way, the "moon" you see is actually the lunate bone abnormally turned from its normal alignment in the wrist.

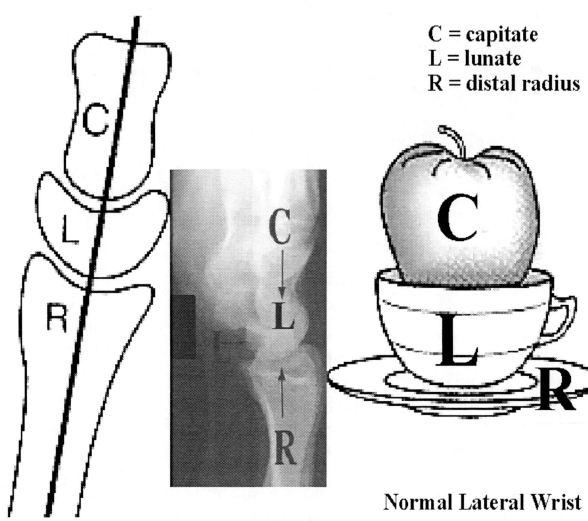

C = capitate
L = lunate
R = distal radius

Normal Lateral Wrist

Figure B-33

Lunate Dislocation (anterior)

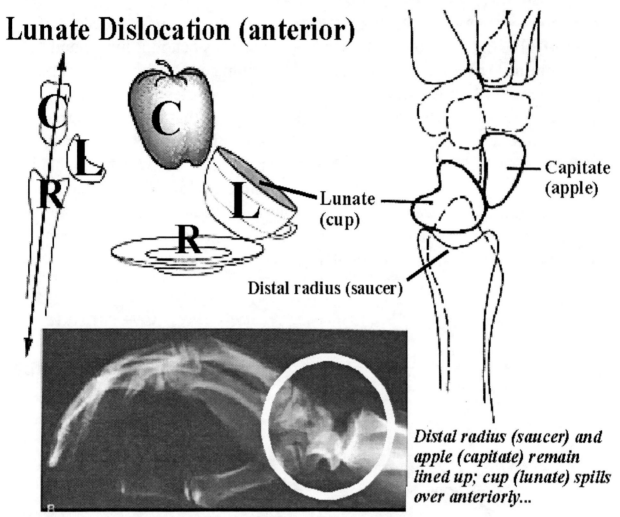

Lunate (cup)

Capitate (apple)

Distal radius (saucer)

Distal radius (saucer) and apple (capitate) remain lined up; cup (lunate) spills over anteriorly...

Figure B-34

If you're interested in differentiating a lunate from a perilunate dislocation, the following analogy may be helpful. On the lateral wrist film, it's easy to trace the outlines of the distal radius, lunate, and capitate. In fact, these bones form a series of shadows that resembles a saucer (distal radius) with a cup sitting on top of it (lunate) and an apple sitting in the cup (capitate) [Figure B-33]. In a

> *REMEMBER* — **You should never see the moon in the wrist; if you do, there is a "lunate bone twist!"**

lunate dislocation, the lunate dislocates anteriorly (towards the palm). The result on the lateral is that the "cup" appears to have spilled over, while the saucer (distal radius) and apple (capitate) remain lined up (Figure B-34). In a

perilunate dislocation, the capitate and remainder of the distal hand bones dislocate posteriorly (away from the palm) from the lunate (Figure B-35). The result on the lateral is that the "apple" is shifted away from the "cup" and "saucer," which remain in alignment.

REMEMBER — A fracture by any other name would look (smell??) just as bad (sweet??)!

With either type of lunate dislocation, the end result is that the lunate becomes "uncovered" and "sticks out" on the lateral — thus, the appearance of the moooooon in the wrist! Realistically, whether or not you remember the difference, the bottom line is simple — if you see the "moon in the wrist," there is a "lunate bone twist." In most cases, that's all you really need to know to invite your friendly local (versus general???) orthopedic specialist to join the party! It is always important to check the alignment of the saucer, cup, and apple,

REMEMBER — In any wrist fracture, always check for carpal dislocation... Do the saucer, cup, and apple line up?

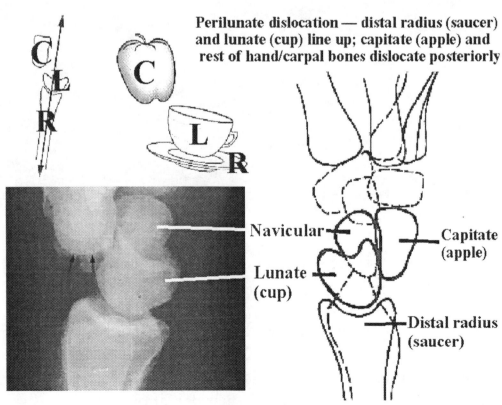

Perilunate dislocation — distal radius (saucer) and lunate (cup) line up; capitate (apple) and rest of hand/carpal bones dislocate posteriorly

Navicular

Capitate (apple)

Lunate (cup)

Distal radius (saucer)

Figure B-35

especially in fractures of the wrist, since the two injuries are commonly associated. A concomitant carpal bone dislocation ("twist") makes a simple fracture (if there is really such a thing) far more complicated.

Fractures of the distal radius are known as **Smith's fractures** or **Colle's fractures**, depending on the direction of displacement of the distal fragment (Figure B-36). In the Smith fracture, the fragment is displaced in a volar direction; in the Colle's fracture, it is dorsally displaced. Is anyone (besides me) confused yet? This is *exactly* why I don't recommend learning eponyms (names adapted from a person's

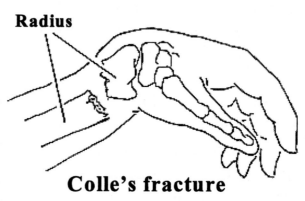

Radius

Colle's fracture

Figure B-36

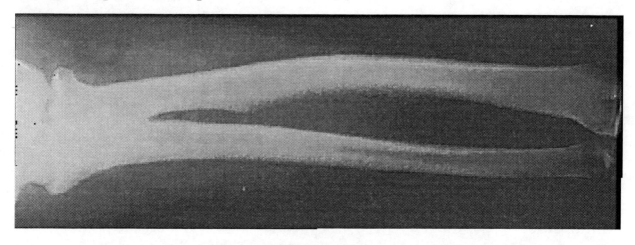

Normal forearm (radius and ulna)

Figure B-37

name) for *any* injury. Rather than try to memorize the names, just make sure you are able to recognize that a fracture exists. The name doesn't really matter as long as you don't miss the fracture! Get two views at right angles to each other to appreciate radial-ulnar deviation as well as displacement in the dorsal-volar plane. Describe *what* you see (e.g., fracture of the distal radius with dorsal displacement of the distal fragment) and you'll always be sure about communicating the appropriate information to your colleagues.

Forearm — The distal forearm is the wrist, and the proximal forearm is the elbow. So, all we really have left are the shafts of the radius and ulna. Guess what? The same rules apply — either they're smooth or they're broken (Figure B-37)! Nothing fancy here...

Elbow — The elbow film is a lot of fun. There are a couple of soft tissue shadows that allow you to call an x-ray abnormal and *never* see a fracture line! This makes sense when we look at the anatomy of the elbow joint. There are two pieces of fat, or fat pads, normally located in the elbow — one in front (**anterior fat pad**) and the other posteriorly (**posterior fat pad**). Fat is very radiolucent and casts a very dark shadow on the film. The anterior fat pad normally lies flat against the anterior border of the distal humerus. Since it's right out there in the open, you'd expect to see it on a

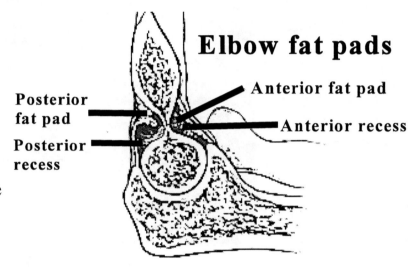

Elbow fat pads

Posterior fat pad

Posterior recess

Anterior fat pad

Anterior recess

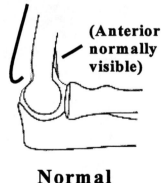

(Posterior normally not seen)

(Anterior normally visible)

Normal

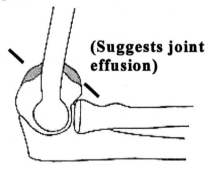

Abnormal = anterior FP "sailed forward" *or* posterior FP visible at all...

(Suggests joint effusion)

Abnormal

Figure B-38

normal lateral elbow film. On the other hand, the posterior fat pad lies in the recess between the lateral and medial portions of the posterior humerus (**olecranon fossa**). Since it's normally obscured by bone on each side, the posterior fat pad is "invisible" to the x-ray beam (Figure B-38).

If fluid (effusion) accumulates within the elbow joint for any reason, it dissects behind both of the fat pads, pushing them away from the bone. The normally flat anterior pad then appears like a sail coming out from the humerus, while the posterior pad becomes visible as a dark shadow directly posterior to the border of the posterior humerus. The presence of *either* of these signs is always abnormal and suggests an elbow joint effusion (Figures B-39, B-40). Thus, our rules:

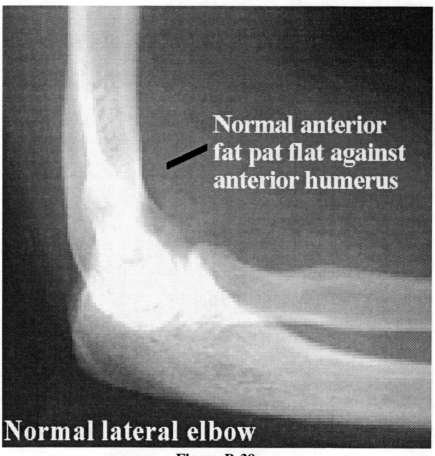

Normal anterior fat pat flat against anterior humerus

Normal lateral elbow

Figure B-39

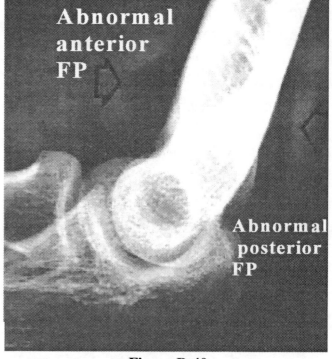

Abnormal anterior FP

Abnormal posterior FP

Figure B-40

BONES-36

- An anterior fat pad flat against the bone is normal.

- An anterior fat pad "sailed out" forward is *always* abnormal.

- A visible posterior fat pad is *always* abnormal.

The **"fat pad sign"** indicates fluid within the elbow joint. It does not tell you what *type of effusion* is present. A common cause of the "fat pad sign" is an occult radial head fracture. These injuries often occur during a fall, hitting the lateral aspect of the elbow. The patient is tender over the radial head in the antecubital fossa. Most times, the fracture itself is not visible on x-ray but bleeding within the joint still occurs. The bloody effusion causes the fat pads to move, and the fat pad sign becomes visible.

Any effusion (e.g., septic arthritis, gout, rheumatoid arthritis) in the elbow joint can lead to a positive fat pad sign, not just fractures of the radial head, though these are the most common cause post-trauma. Injuries that tear the joint capsule, such as elbow fractures or dislocations, *rarely* result in a fat pad sign since the effusion is no longer contained within the tense synovial membrane. The fat pad sign is *most* helpful to distinguish an abnormal from a normal elbow where no other x-ray findings are present.

> ### *Rules of the Elbow:*
>
> - **An anterior fat pad flat against the bone is normal.**
>
> - **An anterior fat pad "sailed out" forward is *always* abnormal.**
>
> - **A visible posterior fat pad is *always* abnormal.**

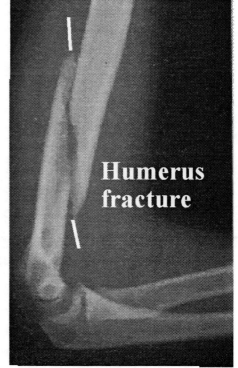

Humerus fracture

Figure B-41

Arm (Humerus) — The distal humerus forms part of the elbow joint, while the proximal end makes up part of the shoulder. The remaining portion of the humerus, the shaft, is easy to make sense out of on x-ray — either the cortex is smooth or the humerus is broken! Remember that the radial nerve wraps around the midportion of the humerus. Fractures in this area may damage the nerve, leading to wrist drop (Figure B-41).

Shoulder, clavicle, and acromioclavicular (AC) joint — One of the most common errors I have seen is obtaining *acromioclavicular (AC) joint* films when the patient had a *shoulder* injury and vice versa. First of all, let's get the anatomy straight. Follow the diagram below and locate your sternoclavicular joint. This one is pretty easy, right? Now, move laterally along the clavicle until it stops — this point is the AC joint! It's *not* the shoulder as many people erroneously think. The shoulder is the *next* bump laterally and

> *REMEMBER* — Shoulder and AC joints are distinct both anatomically and clinically; each requires a very different x-ray technique!

inferiorly. The reason I'm being so darn picky about this difference is because the shoulder and the AC joint films are done differently. If you obtain a shoulder film when the patient has an AC joint problem, there's a good chance you'll miss a partial separation (see below).

Guess what? Either the clavicular cortex is smooth or the bone is broken (Figure B-42)! Just as we've said for *every* other bone so far (and will continue to say). By itself, this fracture is painful and bothersome. Underlying damage from the fracture fragments (e.g., pneumothorax, subclavian vessel tear), however, can be life-threatening. The middle one-third is the most commonly fractured portion of the clavicle.

> *REMEMBER* — Always look for underlying pneumothorax and pleural effusion in patients with clavicle fractures...

The lateral end of the clavicle articulates with the acromion process of the scapula, forming the **acromioclavicular** or **AC joint**. This joint is supported by two ligaments (**acriomioclavicular ligament** and **coracoclavicular ligament**) and the joint capsule (Figure B-43). Various types of injuries, such as blocking during a football game, can tear any or all of the supporting tissues, leading to an AC separation ("separated shoulder").

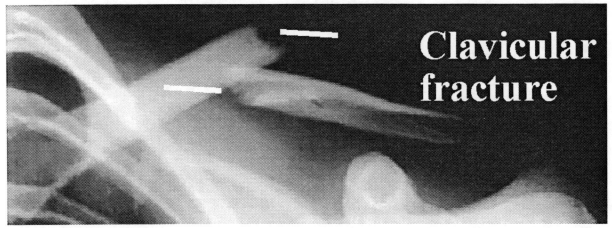

Figure B-42

If all three ligaments are completely torn, the

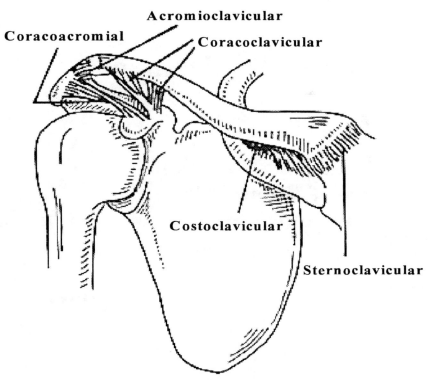

Normal AC joint ligaments
Figure B-43

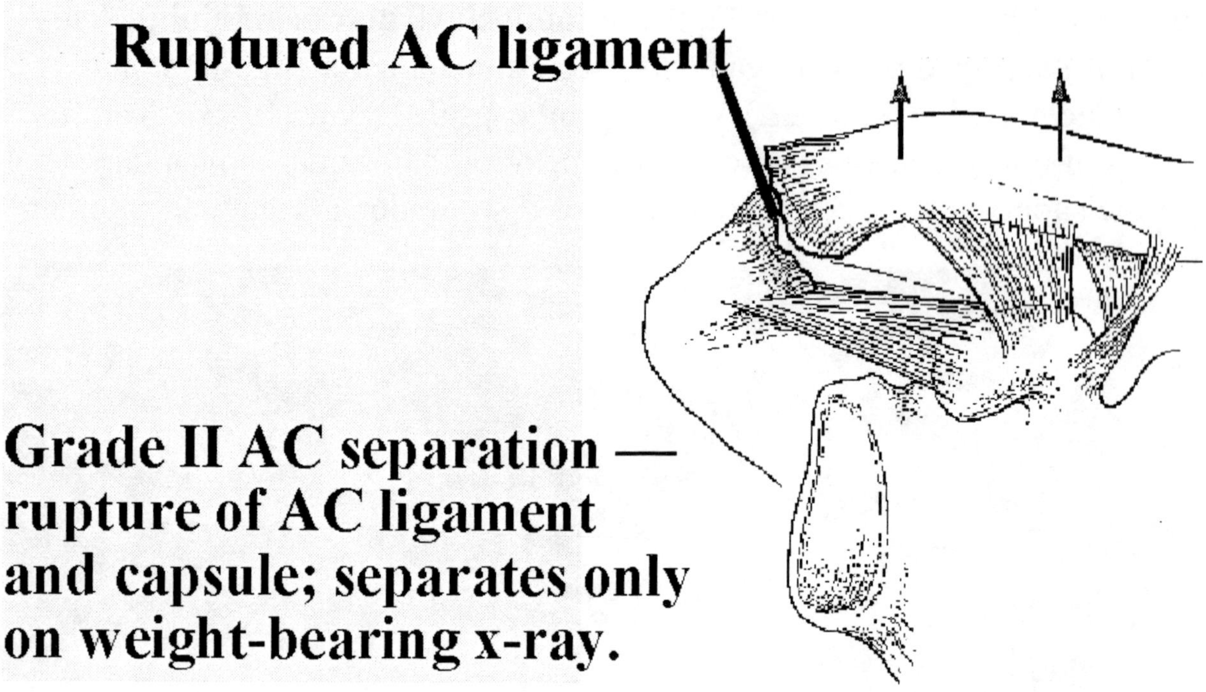

Ruptured AC ligament

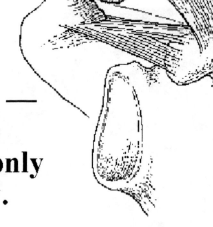

Grade II AC separation — rupture of AC ligament and capsule; separates only on weight-bearing x-ray.

Figure B-44

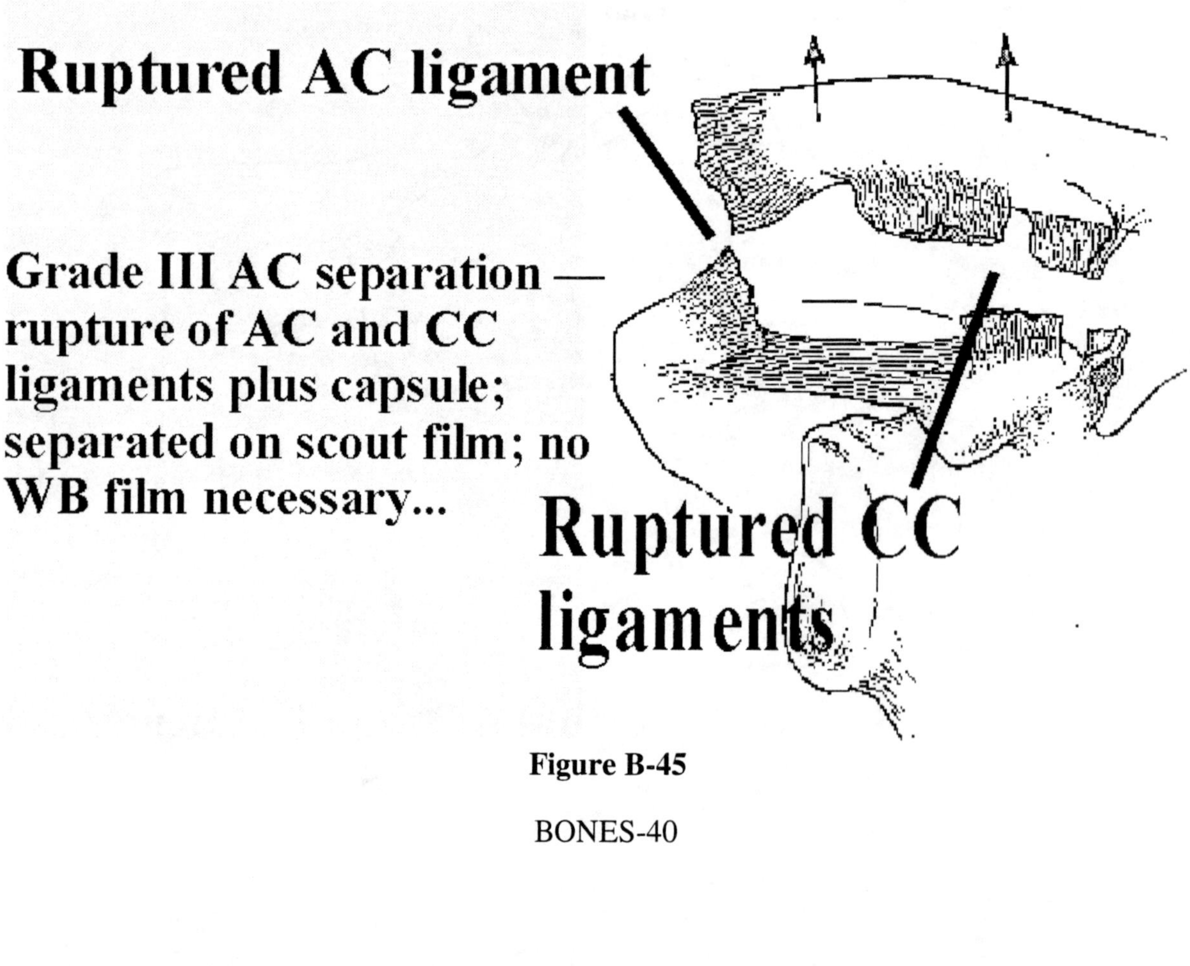

Ruptured AC ligament

Grade III AC separation — rupture of AC and CC ligaments plus capsule; separated on scout film; no WB film necessary...

Ruptured CC ligaments

Figure B-45

clavicle moves superiorly away from the acromion creating a visible and palpable deformity. If any of the ligaments remain intact, the separation is less than complete.

The radiographic degree of separation is ranked by grades, with **Grade III** being *complete* separation *prior to* weight bearing, and **Grade I** indicating *no* separation with weight bearing. **Grade II** results in some separation, but *only* with weight-bearing. The anatomical causes and prognostic implications for each grade of AC separation are different. Thus, weight-bearing films are necessary in all but the most obvious Grade III injuries (Figures B-44, B-45, B-46). They are *essential* to diagnose Grade II injuries and differentiate them from Grade III injuries [T.H. Berquist, Imaging of Orthopedic Trauma and Surgery, Saunders 1986, p. 549]. The radiographer obtains films with and without the patient holding light weights (2.5 - 5 pounds) on the affected side. In a partial tear, the weight causes the joint to separate, as compared to

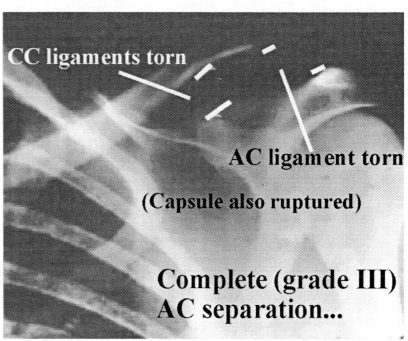

Figure B-46

the non-weight-bearing view. Because the weights are so light, the chances of worsening the injury are very slim. If a complete separation is visible on a non-weight-bearing film, stress (weight-bearing) films are not necessary.

CLASSIFICATION	X-RAY FINDINGS	PROGNOSIS
Grade I — ligament sprain; a few ligament fibers torn	Normal	No instability; excellent
Grade II — rupture of the capsule and acromioclavicular ligaments	Joint wide; clavicle may be slightly elevated	90% recover, 10% may require surgery for persistent symptoms
Grade III — rupture of capsule, acromioclavicular ligaments, and coracoclavicular ligaments	Elevated clavicle, increased coracoclavicular distance (distal clavicle "juts into the air")	Requires surgery for internal fixation; 80% have good result, 20% require reoperation

The normal shoulder joint contains, in addition to the bony structures, numerous ligaments and tendons that are not usually visible on plain x-rays.

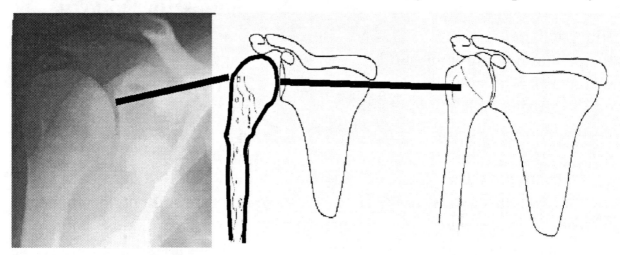

Normal humerus head looks like a "walking stick..."
Figure B-47

Occasionally, abnormal calcification due to injury or inflammation may be noted. The width of the space between the humeral head and the glenoid fossa remains relatively constant from top to bottom on the AP film. The head of the humerus in a normal AP film is asymmetrical, and has been likened to a "walking stick" (Figure B-47).

If the patient suffers a *posterior dislocation*, the humeral head internally rotates and then moves posteriorly. Rather than appear like a "walking stick," the internal rotation causes the head to look more symmetrical, much like a "lightbulb." It is very difficult to see this injury without special films, but widening of the gleno-humeral space is common and relatively easy to notice. Fortunately, most shoulder dislocations are anterior, anterior-inferior, or anterior-superior. And, they're real easy to see — when the humeral head no longer "lives" in the glenoid fossa, the shoulder's dislocated (Figure B-48)!

> **REMEMBER — Most shoulder dislocations are anterior; most hip dislocations are posterior...**

About the only time you will see a posterior dislocation is following a grand mal seizure or electrocution. Massive contractions of the thoracic muscles literally pull the humeral head out of socket. These injuries are often bilateral — if not, comparison views of the uninjured shoulder may be very helpful in finding a posterior dislocation (Figure B-49).

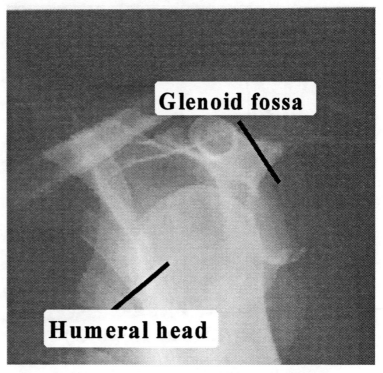

Anterior dislocation — "The humerus doesn't live here anymore!"
Figure B-48

Overlap of humeral head on glenoid fossa...

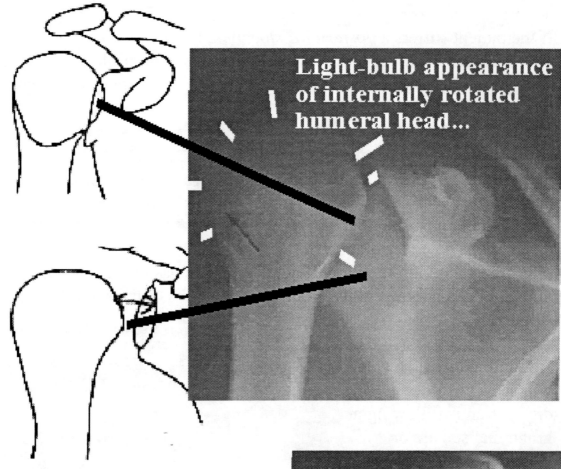

Light-bulb appearance of internally rotated humeral head...

Widening of joint space due to internal rotation...

(Note slightly asymmetrical "walking stick" appearance of normal humeral head...)

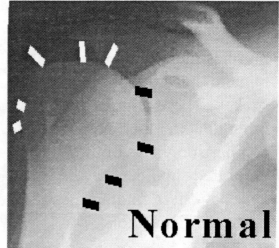

Normal

Figure B-49

THE PELVIS AND HIPS

Pelvis — Pelvic fractures are potentially deadly because they cause internal bleeding. In addition, the underlying gastrointestinal and genitourinary structures are easily damaged. Despite the fact that these fractures are orthopedically exciting (MOTs), the first priority is *always* the ABCs (airway, breathing, circulation). Pelvic fractures are a common cause of hypotension after trauma. Many Emergency Departments routinely obtain a portable AP pelvis film on all shocky or unconscious trauma victims.

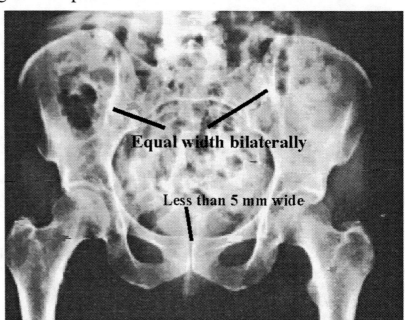

The normal pelvis resembles a well-dressed animal... note the head, the ears, the bowtie, and the earrings! Silly, but this mnemonic forces you to follow the outlines of the entire pelvis so you don't miss a subtle abnormality (Figure B-50). The sacroiliac joint width should be equal on both sides, and the pubic symphysis should be no wider than 5 mm. As you

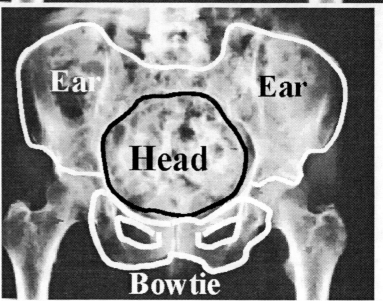

Normal Pelvis X-Ray

Figure B-50

follow the bony cortices, recall that the pubic symphysis is anterior. The rami ("bowtie") form a set of rings. Thus, injury to the superior ramus almost always affects the inferior ramus on the same side as well (Figure B-51). Remember: "When there's one (fracture), look for two...one fractured ramus simply won't do!"

Remember also that the normal patient has stool in the bowel — sometimes it overshadows the bones. Get used to looking at films where the patient has *not* received a bowel prep beforehand — very few sick or injured people have the foresight to clean out their colons for you prior to presenting for care!

Pelvic Film Rules:

- **Sacroiliac joint width equal on both sides.**

- **Pubic symphysis no wider than 5 mm.**

- **Head, ears, bowtie, and earrings are all smooth.**

- **When there's one (fracture), look for two — one fractured ramus simply won't do!**

Hips — The hip joint is the point of articulation of the proximal femur and the acetabulum. Hip fractures are distinguished by their anatomic location (Figures B-52, B-53). The location of the fracture determines, to a great extent, the necessary treatment.

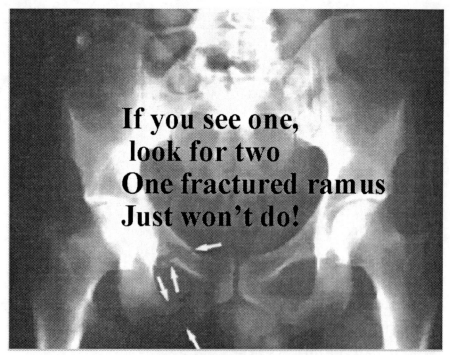

Figure B-51

For example, a patient with a fracture anywhere from the midfemoral neck to the head will likely require joint replacement. The reason? The proximal femur has a poor independent blood supply and avascular necrosis of the femoral head and neck is common. More distal fractures often respond well to orthopedic "nailing" (compression screws) [Figure B-54]. Clinically, shortening and external rotation of the affected extremity are present.

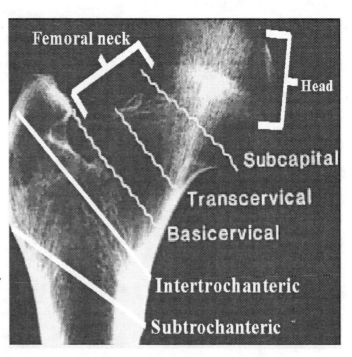

Figure B-52

Hip dislocations usually occur during motor vehicle accidents where the knee is driven into the dashboard (Figure B-55). Forces are directed posteriorly, leading to posterior hip dislocation. Anterior dislocation of the hip is extremely *rare*; posterior dislocation is far more common. The principle of making sense out of the film here is the same as in the shoulder — when the femoral head no longer "lives" in the acetabulum, there's a posterior dislocation. Time to call the Femoral Relocation Service!!

I strongly recommend obtaining bilateral hip films, especially in

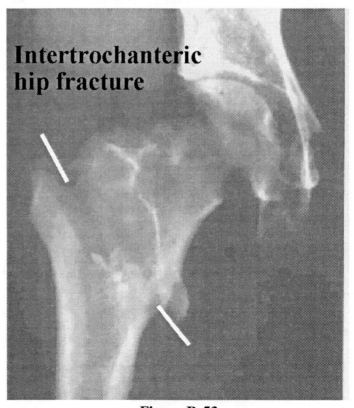

Figure B-53

the geriatric patient. Despite the fact that some hip fractures are quite obvious, an equal number are incredibly subtle. By using the other side (assuming it's uninjured) as a "normal" comparison, subtle fractures may become more obvious (Figure B-56).

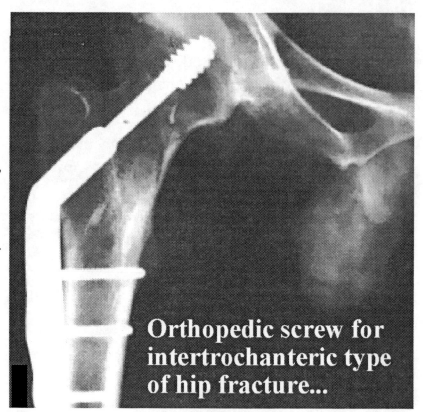

Orthopedic screw for intertrochanteric type of hip fracture...

Figure B-54

FRIENDLY HINT — Get bilateral hip films or a supine pelvis/hips film so you don't miss subtle fractures!

REMEMBER — The most common hip dislocation is posterior; the most common shoulder dislocation is anterior...

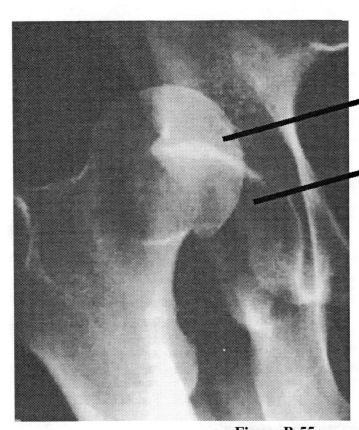

— Femoral head

Acetabulum

**Posterior Hip
Dislocation (most
common)**

Figure B-55

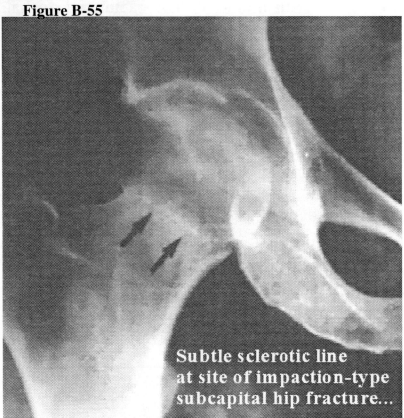

**Subtle sclerotic line
at site of impaction-type
subcapital hip fracture...**

Figure B-56

THE LOWER EXTREMITY

Thigh (Femur) — The femur is the largest and strongest bone in the body. Proximally, it forms the hip joint (along with the pelvic bones) while distally it is the superior portion of the knee. Fractures of the femoral shaft, like those of the pelvis, are also potentially life-threatening. Geometrically, the volume of the thigh space may

> *REMEMBER* — **Femur fractures are associated with significant internal bleeding, regardless of the external appearance of the patient's thigh...**

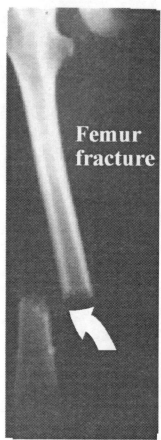

Femur fracture

Figure B-57

accommodate several units of blood *without* any perceptible change in shape to the examiner. Assume any patient with a femoral shaft fracture has lost at least two or three units of blood *per fracture* into the thigh. Again, there's nothing special about finding a fracture of the shaft — and you already know the rule (Figure B-57).

Knee — The knee is a complex joint that is frequently injured. Despite this, the majority of knee x-rays we get are normal. The reason — most injuries involve the nonbony structures (menisci, cruciate or collateral ligaments). The fibula articulates with the proximal tibia and is not functionally part of the knee joint (Figure B-58).

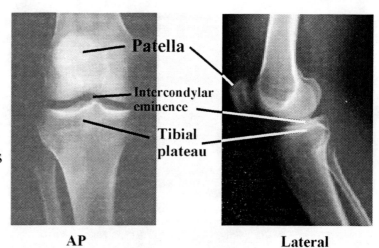

Patella

Intercondylar eminence

Tibial plateau

AP

Lateral

**Normal knee X-ray
Figure B-58**

The patella is a major contributor to the integrity of the knee joint, as well as to leg motion. It is the largest sesamoid bone in the body and lies in the extensor tendon originating in the quadriceps femoris muscles and inserting on the tibial tubercle (Figure B-59). Why the anatomy lesson, you say? Simple — if the patella is fractured there is almost *always* disruption of the extensor tendon (Figure B-60). On the other hand, if the patella is simply dislocated, it's a relatively minor (but painful) injury. The patella *cannot* dislocate superiorly. Clinically, if you palpate the patella in a location more superior than usual, there has almost always been a rupture of some portion of the extensor tendon.

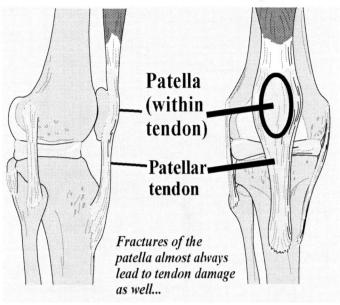

Patella (within tendon)

Patellar tendon

Fractures of the patella almost always lead to tendon damage as well...

Figure B-59

The distal femur rests atop the proximal tibia on the **tibial plateau**. This is also a very important location because the plateau is the major weight-bearing structure of the leg. There are two bony"bumps" called the **intercondylar eminences** (Figure B-61). I call these "Mount Tib" and "Mount Fib." And the rule for this

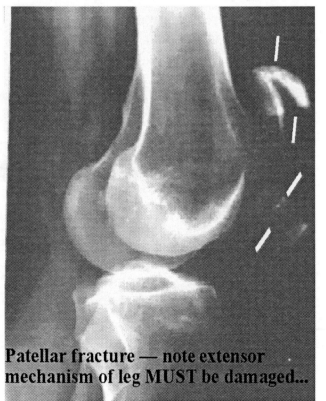

Patellar fracture — note extensor mechanism of leg MUST be damaged...

Figure B-60

portion of the knee is: "You should never see a river between Mount Tib and Mount Fib. If you do, within a fracture lives..." Meaning??? Some tibial plateau fractures are easily seen. Others are more subtle. Often, the fracture line involves the region between the intercondylar eminences, leading to a small radiolucent line between them. The line may or may not run to the edge of the cortex, depending on the severity of the injury and the patient's position. If you see this line ("river") there's a strong likelihood of a tibial plateau fracture (Figure B-62).

> ***REMEMBER*** — "You should never see a river between Mount Tib and Mount Fib. If you do, within a fracture lives..."

> ***REMEMBER*** — Fractures of the patella potentially compromise the quadriceps tendon and the ability to extend ones' leg.

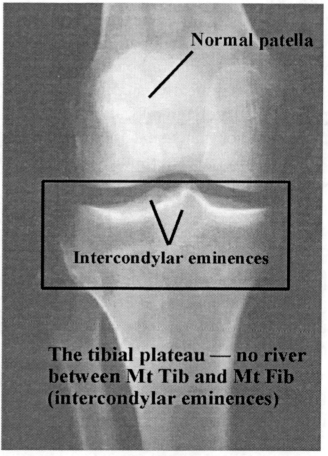

Normal patella

Intercondylar eminences

The tibial plateau — no river between Mt Tib and Mt Fib (intercondylar eminences)

Figure B-61

Leg — The bones of the leg are the fibula and the tibia. Proximally, they form the knee while distally, they form a large part of the ankle mortise (see below). Guess what? You can break the tib, you can break the fib, or you can break *both* the tib and the fib (Figure B-63)!

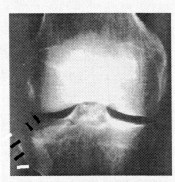

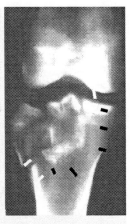

Tibial Plateau Fractures

"You should never see a river between Mount Tib and Mount Fib. If you do, within a fracture lives..."

Figure B-62

Usually, these fractures aren't subtle. The typical boot-top fracture in a skier happens when the ski and boot stop suddenly, but the rest of the skier keeps going — both the distal tibia and fibula are "snapped off" against the movement-resistant boot top.

An easily-missed leg injury is a spiral fracture of the proximal fibula resulting from a sprained ankle. Think about the mechanism of injury — the foot is inverted (turned or twisted inward) for this injury to occur. As the patient's weight moves laterally, a torsion (twisting) force passes up the fibula from the lateral malleolus. To avoid missing this fracture, always check for posterior calf tenderness in all patients with ankle injury, especially involving the lateral malleolus (hyperinversion sprain) [Figure B-64]. In addition, an inversion injury can avulse the peroneus brevis tendon at its point of attachment to the base of the fifth metatarsal (Figure B-65). As in the hand, all you'll see on the x-ray is the bony fragment. During triage, check for tenderness at the base of the fifth toe — if present, get a foot film as well as an ankle film.

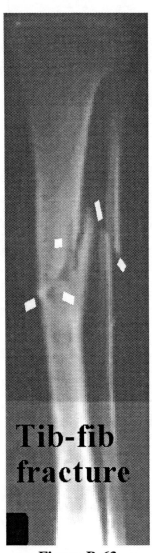

Tib-fib fracture

Figure B-63

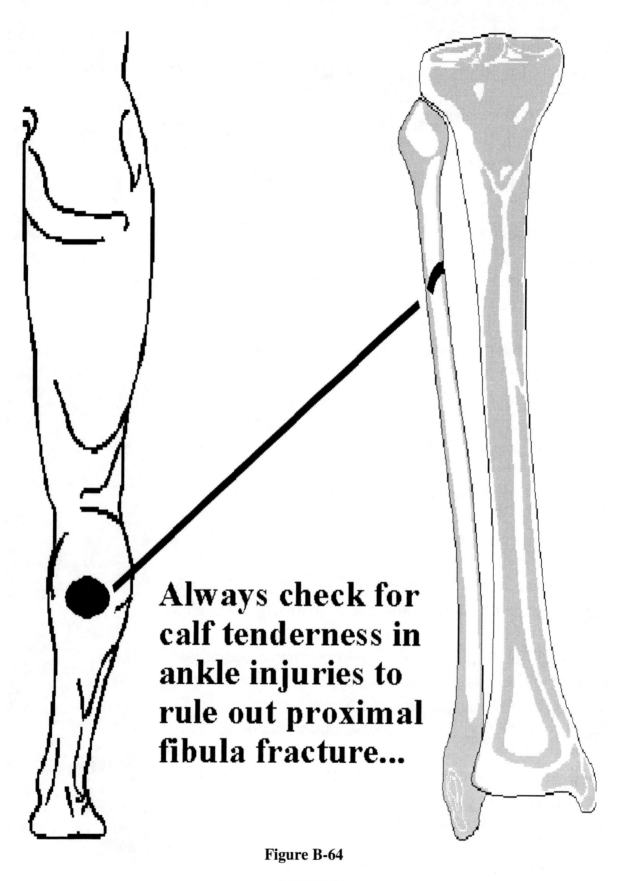

Always check for calf tenderness in ankle injuries to rule out proximal fibula fracture...

Figure B-64

BONES-54

Peroneus brevis tendon avulsion

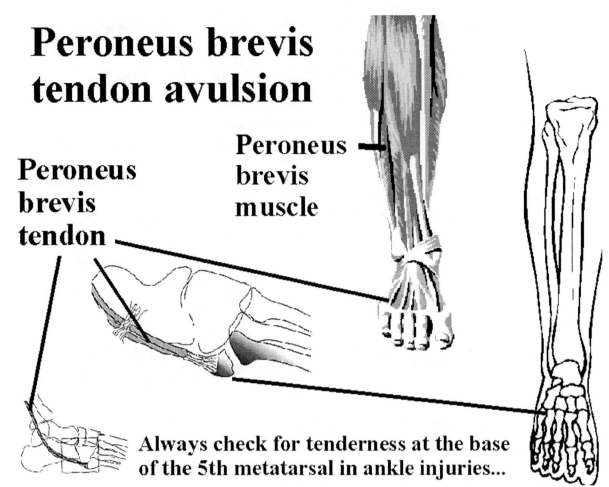

Peroneus brevis tendon

Peroneus brevis muscle

Always check for tenderness at the base of the 5th metatarsal in ankle injuries...

Figure B-65

Ankle and foot — The distal tibia terminates at the medial malleolus while the distal fibula ends at the lateral malleolus. Both articulate at the ankle with the talus. Several ligaments lend security and support to the ankle joint. This important junction is also called the **ankle mortise** (Figure B-66). The most common ankle injury is a sprain, due to either

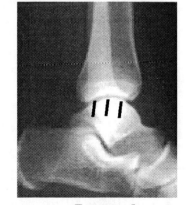

AP   Lateral

Normal ankle film — lines indicate ankle mortise area.

Figure B-66

hyperinversion (turning inward; most common) or hypereversion (turning outward; less common but more serious). Unless there is an accompanying fracture, the plain ankle x-ray is normal, even with a severe sprain. Sometimes, clinicians will do a **stress view** to look for widening of the ankle mortise, indicating ligament instability. Experts disagree as to the value of these films; few Radiology Departments routinely obtain ankle stress film.

There has been much debate concerning whether or not to obtain ankle films for an apparent clinical sprain. Though far from resolved, here are my personal guidelines for ankle injuries:

- If there's bony tenderness over the ankle mortise, get an ankle film.

- If there's also calf tenderness, get a tib-fib film as well.

- If there's also tenderness at the base of the fifth toe, get a foot film, too.

ANKLE TRIAGE TIPS:

- **If there's bony tenderness over the ankle mortise, get an ankle film.**

- **If there's also calf tenderness, get a tib-fib film as well.**

- **If there's also tenderness at the base of the fifth toe, also get a foot film.**

Isolated calcaneal fractures are unusual unless the patient directly kicked a solid object, such as a cement stair or the gate of a pickup truck. Most calcaneal fractures occur after falls. In this case, you *must* look for associated injuries. As the patient hits, the knees typically bend and the trunk arches forward

REMEMBER — **Always look for associated injuries when a patient fractures the calcaneus during a fall...**

(hyperflexion). The result — potential knee and vertebral column injuries (especially compression fractures).

Sometimes you can suspect a cortical compression of the calcaneus even *without* any visible fractures. Draw a line from the posterior aspect ("back bump") of the calcaneus to the highest midpoint ("middle bump"). Now, draw a second line from the highest midpoint to the highest anterior point ("front bump"). The angle between these lines (**Boehler's angle**) should normally be 30-40 degrees. If less than 30 degrees, suspect an impacted fracture of the calcaneus (Figures B-67, B-68). Also look for a sclerotic (white) line where bone trabeculae have been compressed together.

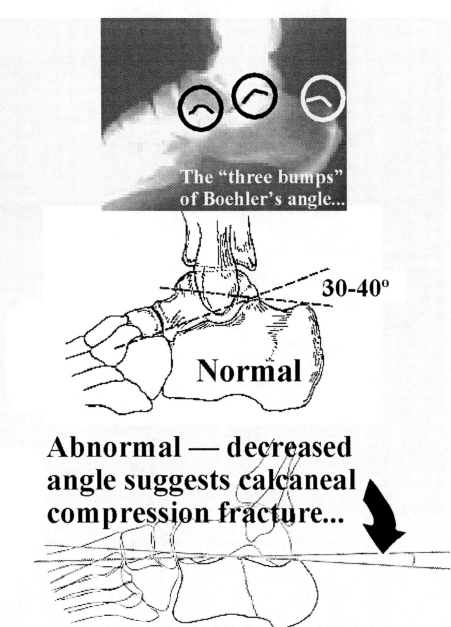

The "three bumps" of Boehler's angle...

30-40°

Normal

Abnormal — decreased angle suggests calcaneal compression fracture...

Figure B-67

The foot bones (tarsals, metatarsals, and phalanges) are relatively straightforward. As in the hand, the bones should line up and the cortices should be smooth (Figure B-69). Otherwise, consider either a dislocation or a fracture.

REMEMBER — The only sign of a calcaneal compression fracture may be a decrease in Boehler's angle.

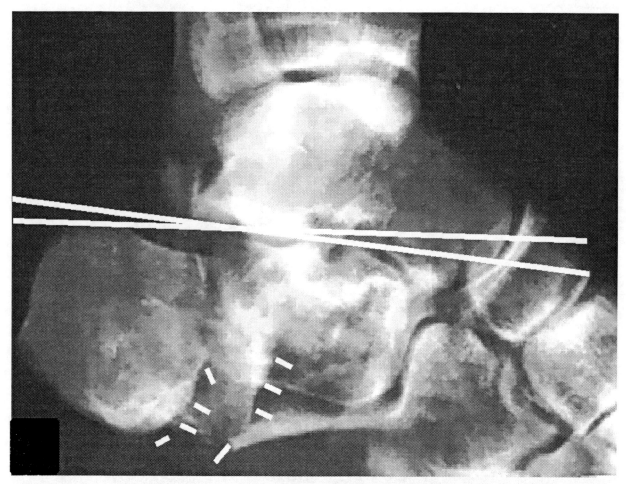

Comminuted calcaneal fracture — note markedly depressed Boehler's angle...

Figure B-68

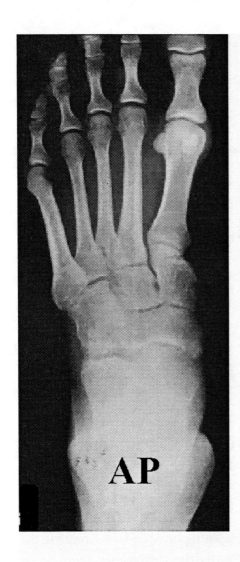

AP

Normal foot X-ray

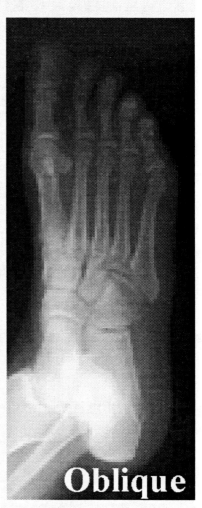

Oblique

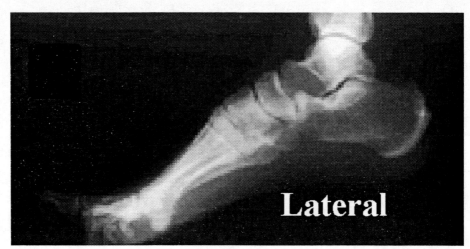

Lateral

Figure B-69

SUMMARY — BONE RULES!

Bones are smooth; when they're not smooth, they're broken...

---

1. Remember that skull and facial x-rays are insensitive indicators of intracranial injury. Evaluate the patient clinically and consider CT scan.

2. When viewing a lateral spine x-ray ask yourself "Do we line up?"

3. Vertebral compression fractures typically result in a trapezoidal shaped vertebral body, with the anterior height significantly (> 1-2 mm) less than the posterior height.

4. Follow the vertebra from anterior to posterior to avoid missing a posterior element injury.

5. The ironic feature of many skull and facial bone series is that they are so difficult to read that other means (e.g., clinical exam, CT scan) are often required to rule out serious intracranial injury.

6. There is no such thing as a "sprained wrist" until you completely rule out a navicular (scaphoid) fracture.

7. Regarding the lateral wrist film: "You should never see the moon in the wrist; if you do, there's a lunate bone twist!"

8. An anterior fat pad flat against the elbow joint is normal; if it's "sailed out," it's always abnormal. A posterior fat pad is *always* abnormal. These abnormal findings indicate the presence of effusion in the joint — a common finding with occult fracture of the radial head.

9. Make sure you know the difference between the AC joint and the shoulder joint!

10. The most common shoulder dislocation is anterior; look for widening of the humeral-glenoid space as a sign of internal rotation and posterior dislocation.

11. Think of the pelvis as a well-dressed animal; remember if one side of the "bow-tie" (e.g., superior ramus) is broken, look for a fracture on the opposite side (e.g., inferior ramus).

12. Consider obtaining bilateral hip films to help see subtle fractures.

13. The most common hip dislocation is posterior.

14. Patients can bleed to death from pelvis or femur fractures.

15. There should never be a river between Mount Tib and Mount Fib.

16. Always check for calf tenderness (fracture of the proximal fibula) and tenderness at the base of the fifth toe (avulsion of peroneus brevis tendon) in a patient with an ankle sprain.

17. Most calcaneal fractures are associated with falls — look for associated injuries.

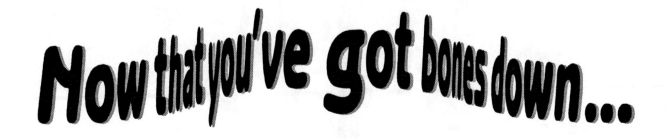

Now that you've got bones down...

It's Gonna Beee a Great Day

Section 4:

Let's Review

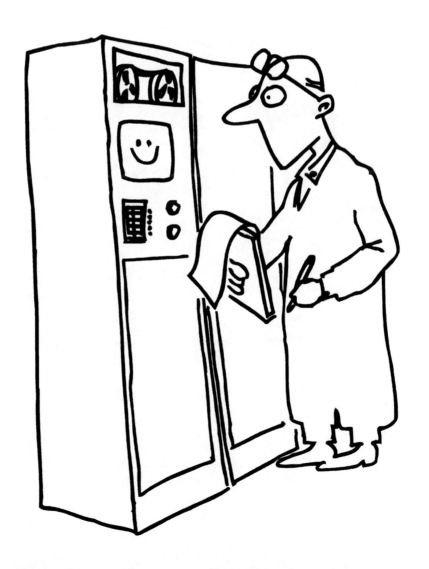

INSTRUCTIONS...

"Let's Review" is a programmed learning review of Sections 1 through 3 of this book. Most of the pages start with a review figure, followed by a table. On the left side of the table are "fill in the blank" questions. The answers are in the right-hand column. To benefit the most, cover the answers while you review the questions first. Then look at the answer to see if you're correct. If not, be sure to understand why. Many of the figures have their original numbers from the first three sections, so you may refer back to salient portions of the book as necessary. Following this portion of the review are several "unknown" x-rays. The instructions given there should be self-explanatory... Have fun!

THE BASICS...

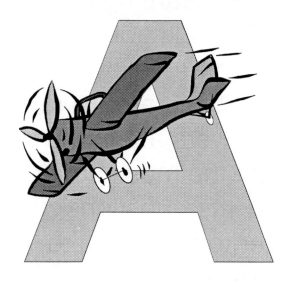

"Plain English"

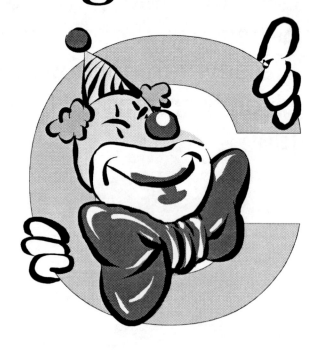

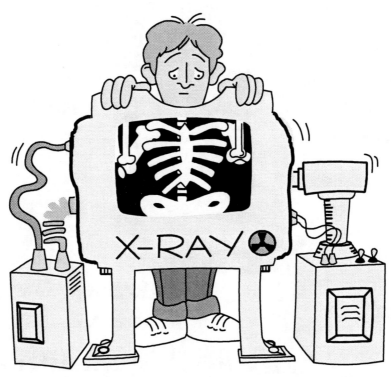

X-rays are fun and easy!!

X-rays are a form of _____ that occupy the upper portion of the electromagnetic spectrum. X-rays are able to _____ materials to a variable degree, depending upon the _____ of the material.	energy penetrate radiographic density

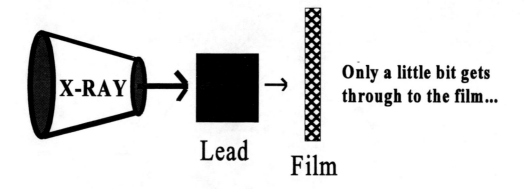

X-RAY → Lead → Film

Only a little bit gets through to the film...

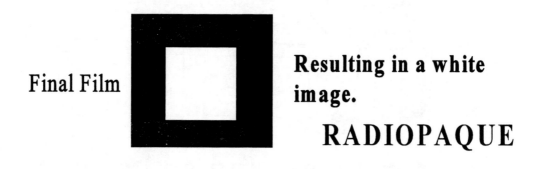

Final Film

Resulting in a white image.

RADIOPAQUE

_____ materials resist the passage of X-rays. As a result, little radiation hits the film plate. The effect is a _____ shadow on the developed film.	Radiopaque white

Radiolucent (air around arm)

Intermediate ("guts" of arm)

Radiopaque (bones)

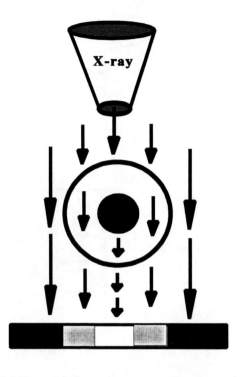

The most radiopaque materials are made of _____. X-rays of these appear _____. Fat is relatively _____ and appears as a _____ shadow. The organs and blood have _____ density and appear as a combination of _____ and _____ "shadows."

metal
white

radiolucent
dark

intermediate

white
dark

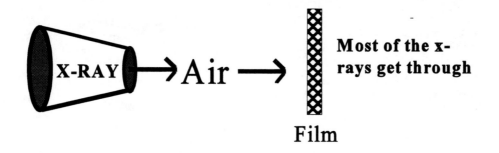

Most of the x-rays get through

Film

Final Film

Resulting in a dark image.

Radiolucent

| _____ objects permit the passage of X-rays to a variable degree, depending on their _____. The greater the number of x-rays that pass through the object, the more radiolucent it is. The most radiolucent substance is _____. Gas appears _____ on the X-ray film. | Radiolucent

density

gas
black (dark) |

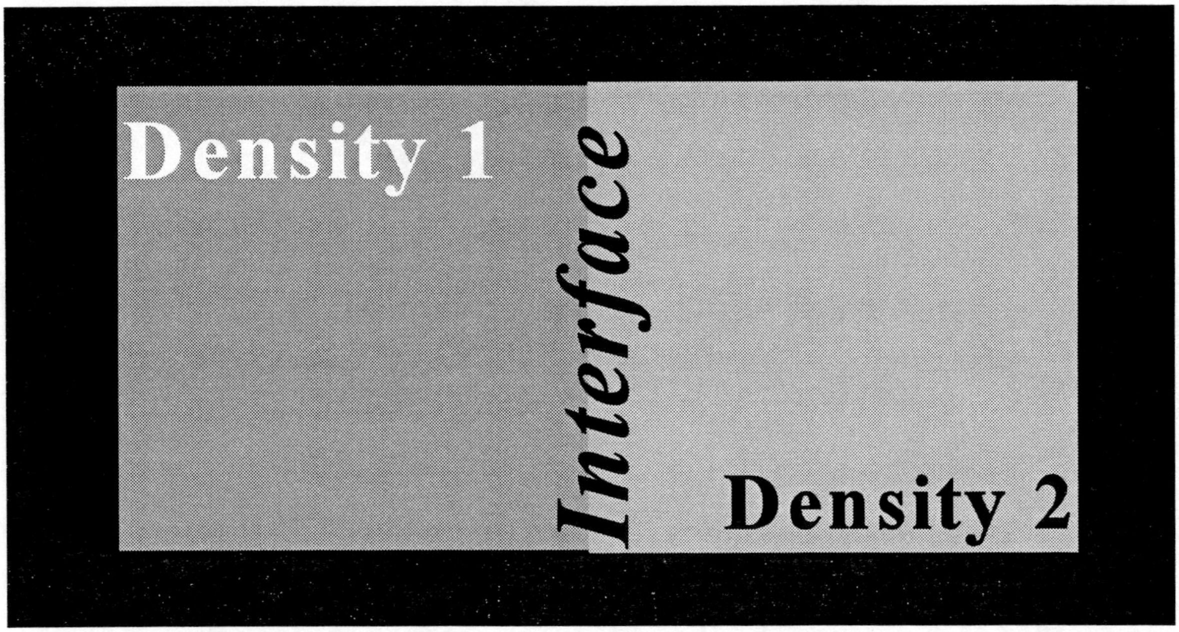

Density 1

Interface

Density 2

Two materials of different density next to each other form a radiographic _____. The greater the difference in density, the _____ the line. Objects of the same density placed next to each other _____ the interface.

interface ("BILL")

sharper

obliterate

The System

- **2 definitions (radiopaque, radiolucent)**

- **3 rules ("BILL")**

- **1 acronym ("I Quit And Wanna Be Free!")**

Approach the x-ray as you would a _____. Perform a quick-scan (primary survey), then analyze the film in more detail using the _____ approach (secondary survey).

patient

"IQAWBF" (I Quit And Wanna Be Free)

Quick Scan
B — bony
S — soft tissue
O — other

The purpose of the "quick scan" is to identify _____ abnormalities. The mnemonic for the quick scan is "BSO" — _____, _____, and _____. Look at the bones for obvious _____. Look at the soft tissues for obvious _____. Look briefly at the organs and make certain things are _____.

obvious

bone, soft tissue
other shadows

deformities

abnormal shadows

where they should be

I Quit And Wanna Be Free!

Identify
Quality
Air shadows
Water shadows
Bone shadows
Funny-looking things

Systematically, _____ the x-ray film. Determine whether the _____ is good enough — are you able to see _____? Then evaluate shadows of _____, _____, and _____. Finally, determine if any _____ are present.

identify

quality

what you need to see

air, water

bone

funny-looking things

Remember, "I _____"	Quit And Wanna Be Free!

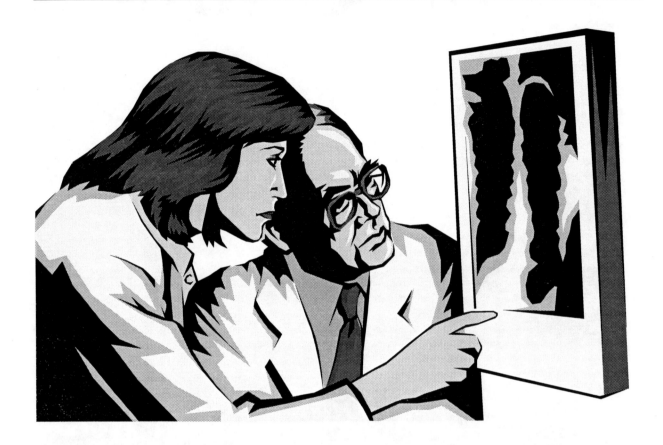

Work together as a team...

An easy way to read x-rays is to compare the film you are studying to the _____.	normal film

The Chest...

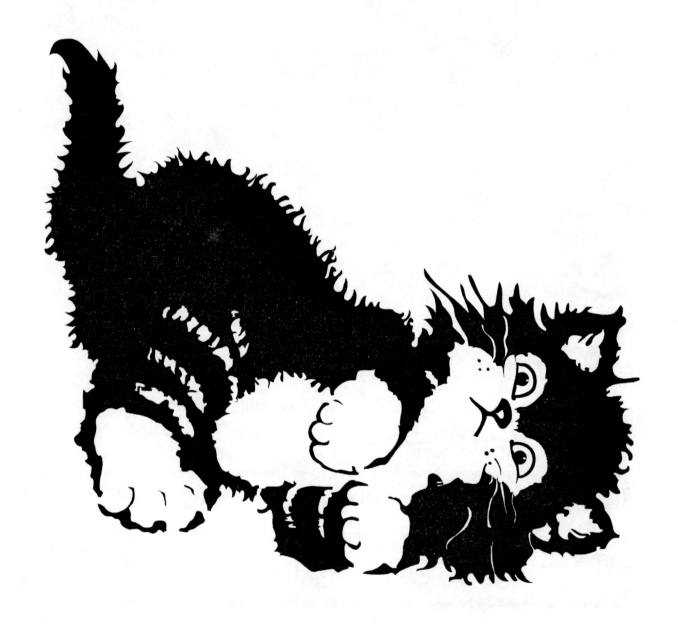

Chest X-Ray Technique

R — Rotation (clavicles and vertebrae form a cross)

I — Inspiration (minimum of 8 ribs visible)

P — Penetration (interspaces visible; thoracic vertebral bodies *not* well-defined)

In a good quality chest film, you should just barely be able to see the _____ of the _____ vertebrae. Both costophrenic _____ should be clear.

intervertebral spaces

thoracic

angles

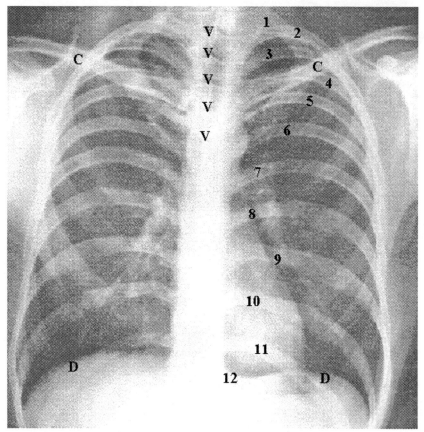

Figure C-1 — Normal Chest Film

The _____ side of the diaphragm shadow should be slightly higher than the left. A "paper-thin" diaphragm indicates _____ in the peritoneal cavity. Lung markings should extend to the _____ of _____ lung fields.

right

free air

periphery
both

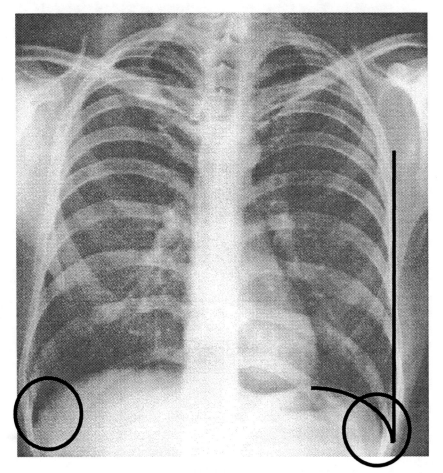

Costophrenic Angles

Figure C-3

With the exception of the heart shadow and the right hemidiaphragm (which is slightly higher than the left), both sides of the chest x-ray should be _____.

symmetrical

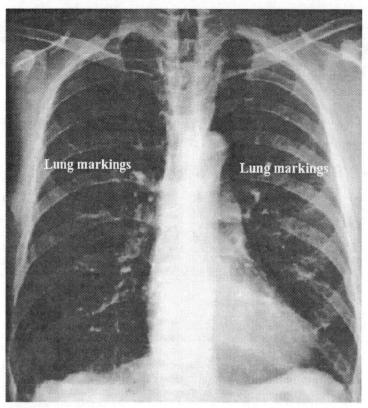

Figure C-6 — Normal lung markings

Bones are _____. An irregularity in the bony cortex suggests a _____.	smooth fracture
Nipple shadows appear as _____ in the lower _____ of the chest x-ray. Breast tissue may cause increased _____ that is usually _____ in nature.	circular densities third radiopacity symmetrical

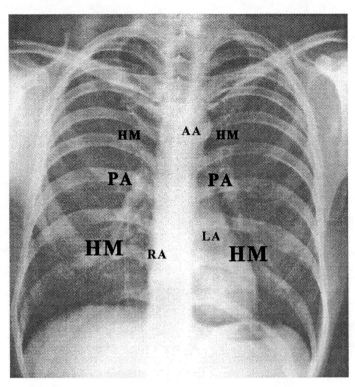

**Pulmonary Arteries (PA)
and Normal Hilar
Markings (HM)**

Figure C-5

The lung shadows represent a combination of alveolar _____, _____, and _____. The carina is where the _____ divides into the right and left _____.

air
blood vessels
lung tissue
trachea

mainstem bronchi

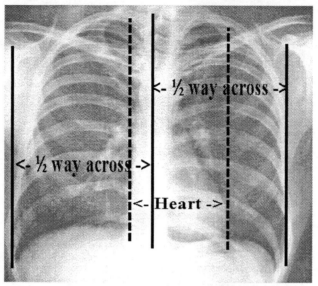

Normal Cardiac Diameter — the heart at its widest point should be less than ½ the distance across the chest at its widest point...

Figure C-4

The normal heart size is less than _____ the distance across the chest area. The hila are where the _____ enter the lungs. In an upright chest x-ray, hilar vascular markings are more prominent in the _____ half of the lung fields due to _____.	half
	pulmonary arteries
	lower
	gravity

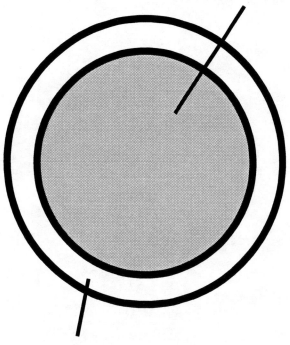

Inside balloon (lung)

Outside balloon (pleura space)

Think of the lung and pleura as two "circus balloons," one inside the other...

Figure C-10A

The pleural cavity is really only a _____. Because the radiographic density of lung tissue and of the pleura is _____, the pleural space _____ visible on normal chest x-rays.	potential space similar is not

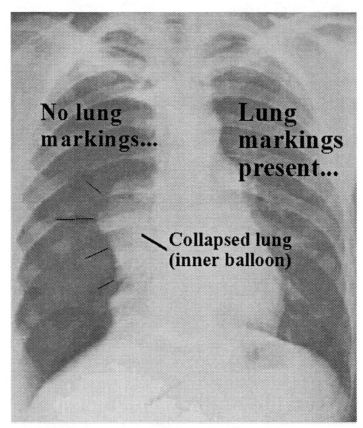

Figure C-11 — Large right pneumothorax

| The lung is totally collapsed in a _____. The involved side appears more _____ than usual and there is an absence of _____. A radiopaque area at the hilum usually represents the _____. | complete pneumothorax

radiolucent (dark)

lung markings

collapsed lung |

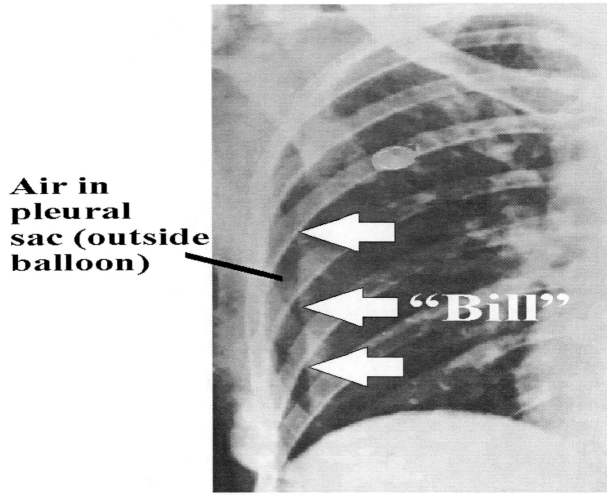

Air in pleural sac (outside balloon)

"Bill"

Figure C-13 — Small pneumothorax (note "Bill")

In tension pneumothorax, the collapsed lung is shifted toward the _____ side. The _____ of the pneumothorax, not its _____, predict the clinical outcome.

opposite

physiologic effects

size

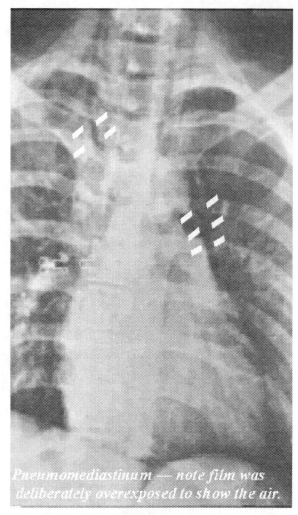

Pneumomediastinum — note film was deliberately overexposed to show the air.

Figure C-14

Air in the mediastinum is called _____.
Causes include

_____, _____,
rupture of the _____,
and _____. Be sure
to exclude concomitant
_____.

pneumomediastinum

trauma, asthma
esophagus
childbirth

pneumothorax

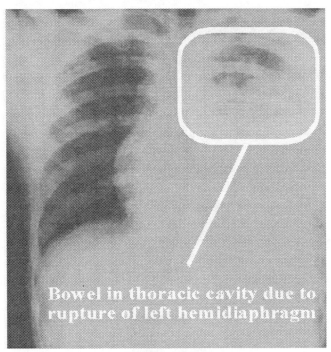

Bowel in thoracic cavity due to rupture of left hemidiaphragm

Figure C-16

The most common cause of a ruptured diaphragm is _____. Most often, the _____ side of the diaphragm is involved. Movement of the stomach and intestines into the chest cavity creates increased _____ in the _____ of the affected side. The diagnostic x-ray finding is the presence of _____ in the chest.

trauma
left

density
lower lung field

loops of bowel

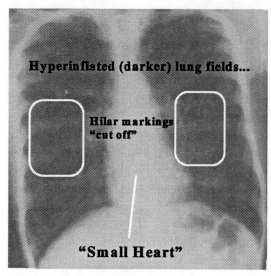

Hyperinflated (darker) lung fields...

Hilar markings "cut off"

"Small Heart"

Results of air trapping from asthma or COPD...

Figure C-17

The primary functional abnormality in both asthma and COPD is _____ to _____ air flow. Air is then _____, leading to _____ of the lungs.	obstruction expiratory trapped hyperinflation
X-ray signs of lung hyperinflation in the PA/AP chest film are _____ of the diaphragms, decreased heart _____, and _____ pulmonary vascular markings.	flattening shadow size decreased

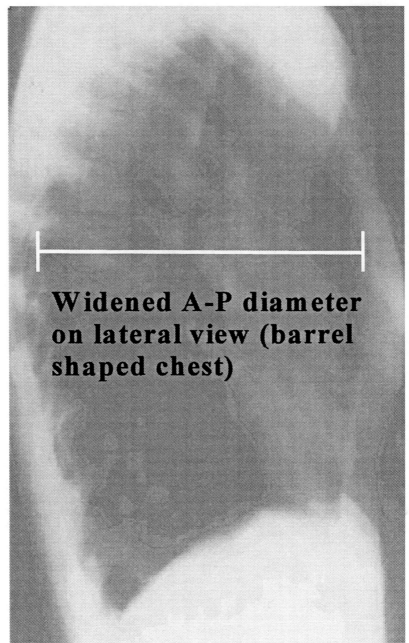

Widened A-P diameter on lateral view (barrel shaped chest)

Figure C-18

Signs of hyperinflation in the lateral chest film include a _____ appearance of the chest.

barrel-shaped

Many asthmatics have normal chest x-rays unless their attacks are _____. Obtain a chest x-ray when the patient fails to respond to _____.

severe

conventional therapy

Most of the time, the chest x-rays of COPD patients are _____, regardless of how they feel. The film is most helpful when it reveals a _____ such as _____ or _____.

abnormal

complication
pneumothorax
pneumonia

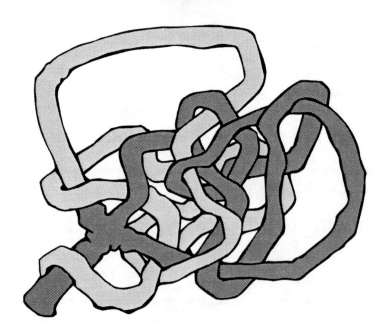

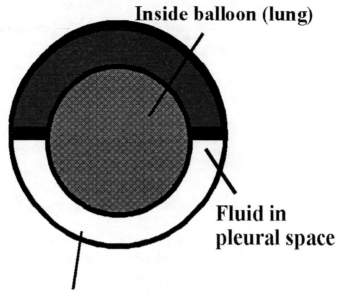

Inside balloon (lung)

Fluid in pleural space

Outside balloon (pleura space)

Pleural Effusion and the Two-Balloon Model

Figure C-19

Irrespective of its composition, fluid has the same _____ on the chest x-ray. A pleural effusion is the abnormal presence of fluid in the _____. Abnormal accumulations of fluid in the lung parenchyma are called _____.	appearance pleural cavity infiltrates

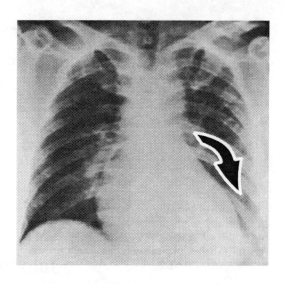

Blunting of left costophrenic angle suggests pleural effusion...

Figure C-21

The earliest chest x-ray sign of a pleural effusion is _____ of the costophrenic angle. This indicates the presence of at least _____ of pleural fluid. The accumulation of more fluid leads to an _____ at the costophrenic angle. The normal lung markings and heart border are _____. With further buildup, the effusion _____, forming a meniscus (level line).	blunting 250 cc upwardly concave density obliterated layers

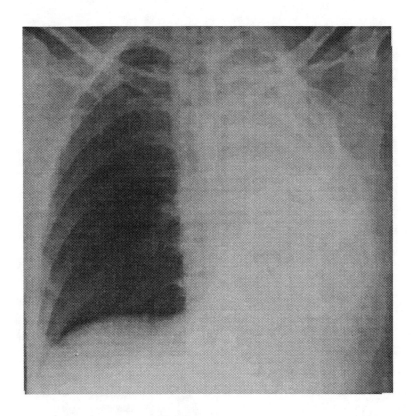

"White-out" of left hemithorax — where is the fluid?
Figure C-26

If a patient with a large pleural effusion lies down, the fluid will flow to _____ portions of the pleural cavity. A supine chest x-ray will show a diffuse _____ representing composite shadows of the _____ and of the _____.

gravity-dependent

density

fluid

lung

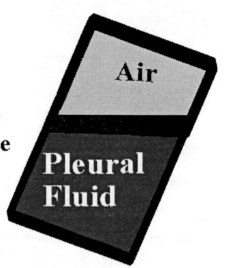

Air

Meniscus

Pleural Fluid

In an upright view, pleural fluid forms an air-fluid level, or a meniscus in the outer balloon.

When the patient moves, so does the fluid...

Air

Pleural Fluid

Figure C-20

To differentiate an infiltrate from a pleural effusion, _____ the patient in a _____ and see if the fluid _____. Fluid that moves with positional changes is most likely due to ——.

place

different position

moves

pleural effusion

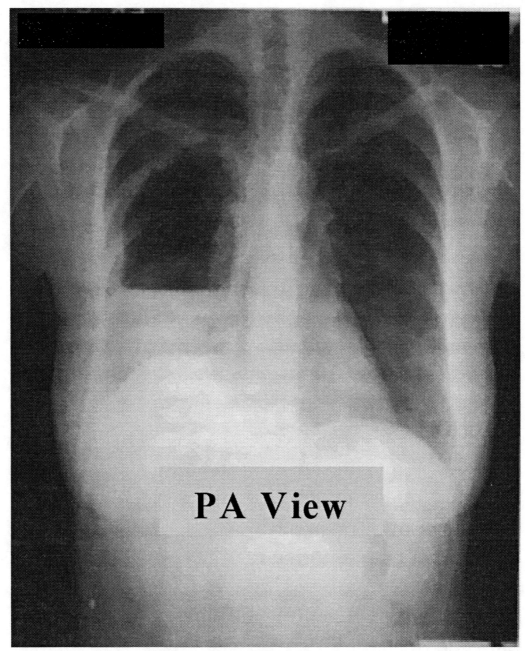

Figure C-24 — Right pleural effusion

| Fluid in the lungs is called an _____. Fluid in the pleural cavity is called a———. | infiltrate

pleural effusion |

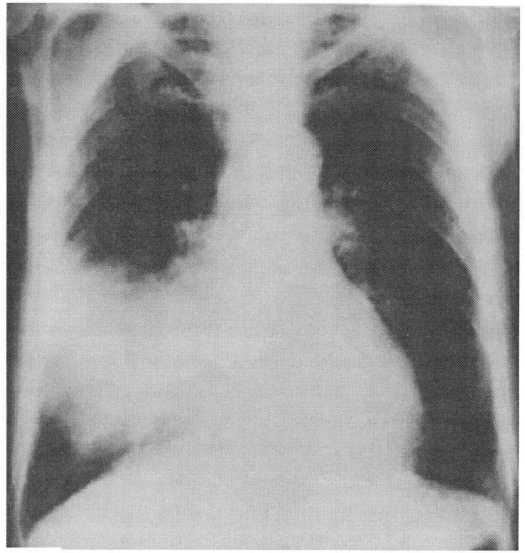

Figure C-29

It is difficult to determine what type of _____ is causing an infiltrate from the x-ray _____. An infiltrate appears as an abnormal _____ density in the lung fields.

fluid

alone

white

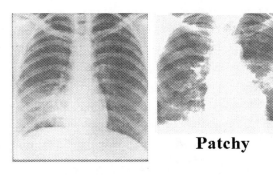

Patchy

Streaky

Diffuse　　**"White-out"**

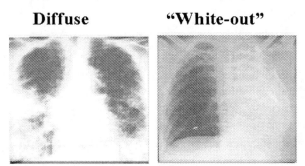

Figure C-28

Linear bands of increased density in the lung fields are called _____ and represent _____ in the _____. Scattered patches of increased fluffy density are called a _____ and represent _____ of the _____ with fluid. A _____ is an infiltrate that involves all of one or both lung fields.	streaky infiltrates fluid interstitial tissue patchy infiltrate filling alveoli white-out

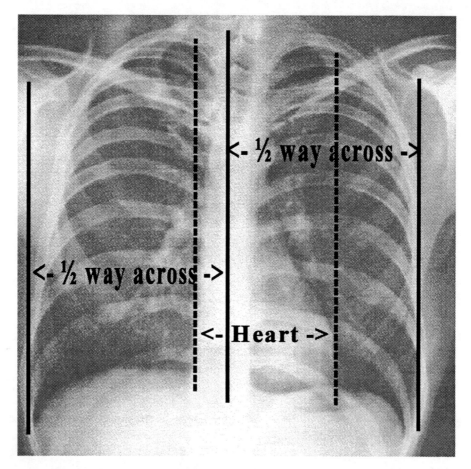

Normal Cardiac Diameter — the heart at its widest point should be less than ½ the distance across the chest at its widest point...

Figure C-35

The normal diameter of the heart is less than _____ the distance from the _____ to the _____.

one-half
rib border
middle of the thoracic vertebrae

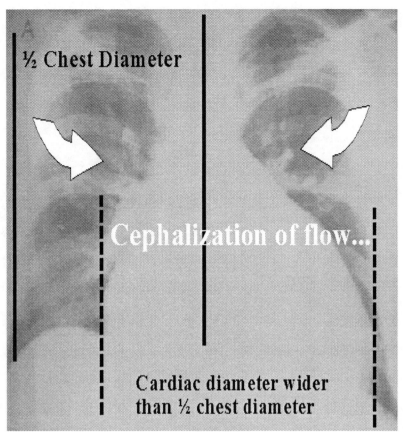

½ Chest Diameter

Cephalization of flow...

Cardiac diameter wider than ½ chest diameter

Figure C-36

The chest x-ray signs of progressive CHF are _____, redistribution of blood to the _____, and a _____ of the hilum, indicating fluid in the _____. As fluid in the alveoli increases, the x-ray shows _____.

cardiomegaly

upper lobes
butterfly appearance

alveoli

snowball-like infiltrates

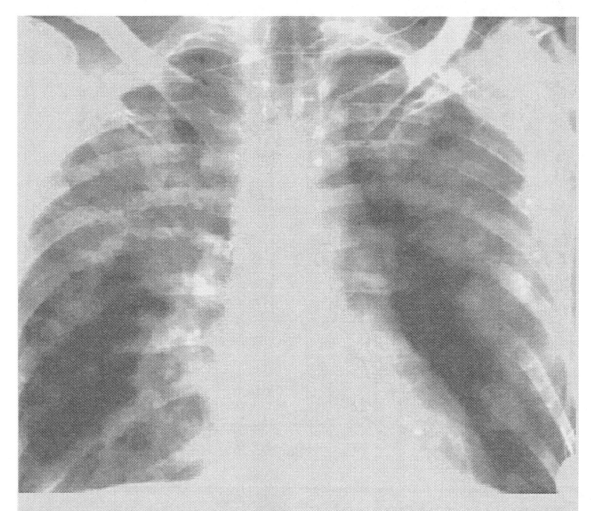

Adult respiratory distress syndrome (ARDS) — note normal heart size and bilateral infiltrates...

Figure C-39

Chest x-ray findings in ARDS include a _____, bilateral _____, and no _____ of blood flow to the upper lobes.

normal-sized heart
infiltrates
redistribution

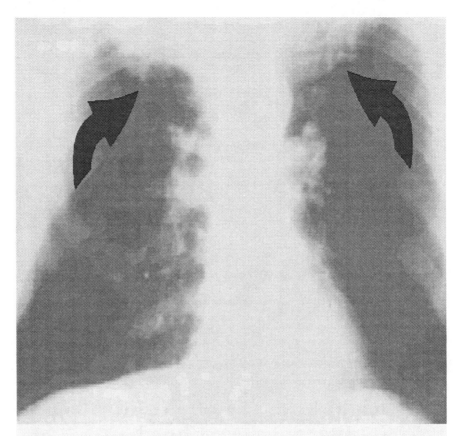

Bilateral upper lobe infiltrates...

Figure C-33

Pneumonia is caused by _____ of the lungs. It appears on x-ray as an _____. Do not attempt to make the _____ of pneumonia based on an _____ alone. Use other _____ as well.

inflammation

infiltrate

diagnosis

x-ray

clinical information

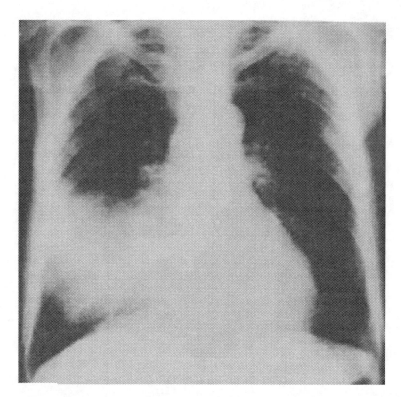

Right Middle Lobe Infiltrate
(obliterates heart border)...

Figure C-31

A right middle lobe or lingular infiltrate obscures the _____, but does not affect the border of the _____. Lower lobe infiltrates obliterate the _____, but spare the _____. Upper lobe infiltrates may obliterate the _____.	heart border diaphragm diaphragm border heart border vertebral shadow

The most common chest x-ray finding in a pulmonary embolism is _____.	a normal film
A bruise to the lung from trauma is called a _____. On x-ray, it appears as an _____ due to _____ into the alveoli and interstitial tissue. This finding may look exactly like the x-ray findings in _____. You cannot tell them apart based on the _____ alone.	pulmonary contusion infiltrate bleeding pneumonia chest x-ray

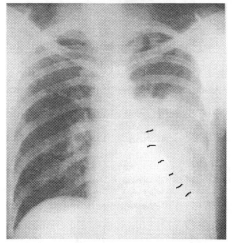

Figure C-34 — Left lower lobe infiltrate (note heart border is clear, but difficult to see because the infiltrate has a similar density...)

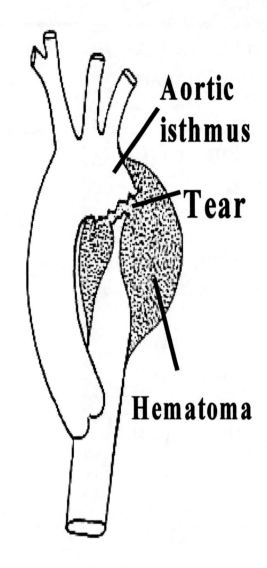

Aortic isthmus

Tear

Hematoma

Figure C-40

5% of patients with acute aortic rupture form a _____ at the site. Ultimately, this _____, leading to exsanguination if not rapidly treated.	hematoma ruptures

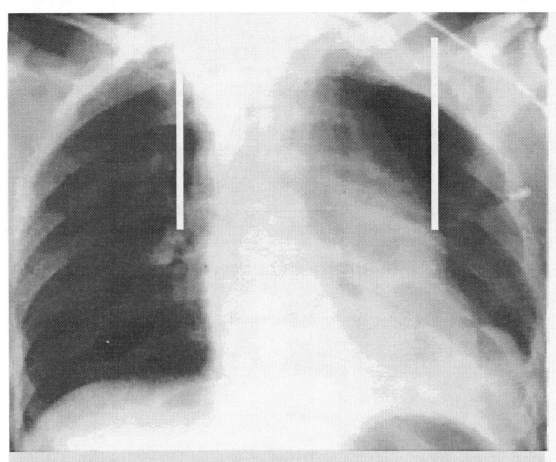

Widening of mediastinum due to aortic trauma...

Figure C-41

Chest x-ray findings associated with rupture of the aorta include _____ of the mediastinum, left-sided _____, obliteration of the _____, and fractures of ribs _____.	widening pleural effusion aortic knob 1-3

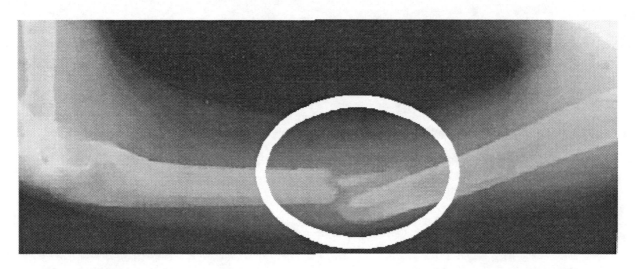

Bones are smooth; when they're not, they're broken

Figure C-42

| Follow the _____ of each rib. The cortical margins should be _____. A _____ in the cortex suggests a fracture. | outlines

smooth
break |

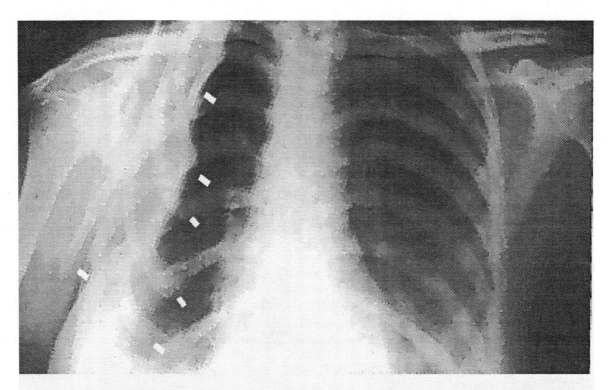

R. sided flail chest due to multiple rib fractures...

Figure C-43

Multiple rib fractures may lead to a condition known as _____. The injured area moves _____ from the normal chest wall. This abnormal movement results in a marked _____ in the effectiveness of ————.

flail chest

in the opposite direction

decrease

breathing

Regarding bony metastases, _____ lesions destroy the bone matrix, resulting in areas of _____ radiographic density. _____ lesions cause overgrowth of _____, leading to _____ radiographic density.

osteolytic

decreased
Osteoblastic

abnormal bone
increased

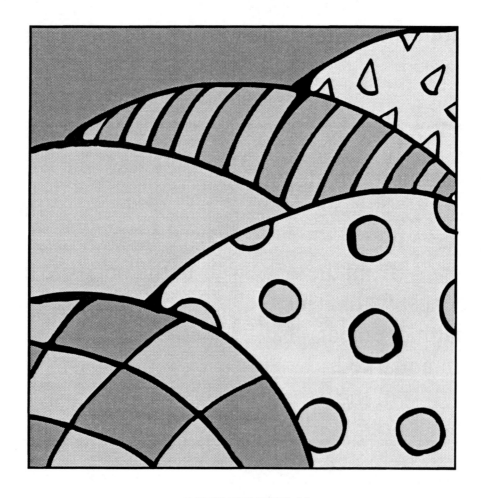

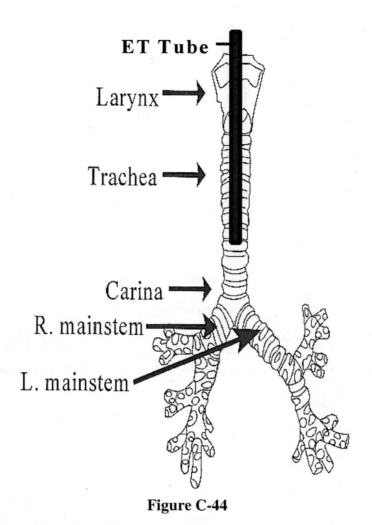

ET Tube

Larynx ➤

Trachea ➤

Carina ➤

R. mainstem ➤

L. mainstem

Figure C-44

The tip of an endotracheal tube should be _____ above the carina. You must _____ the carina in order to determine its position. If you cannot adequately discern the carina, _____.	3-6 cm see repeat the film

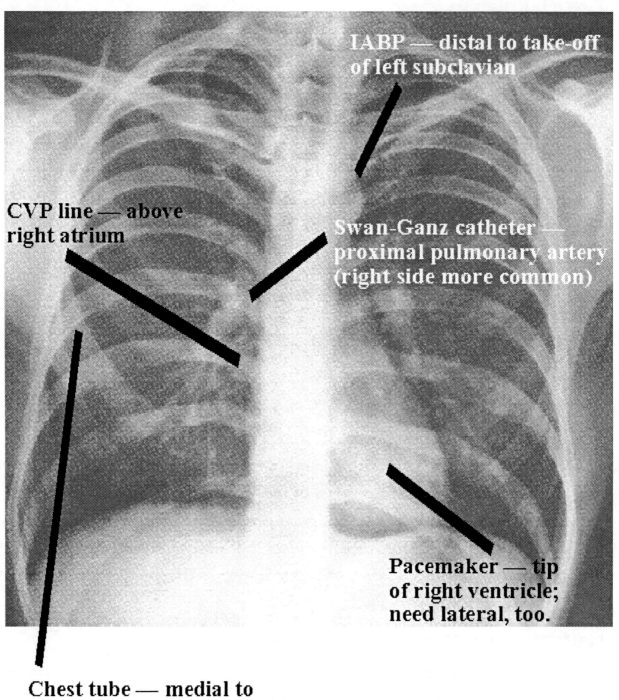

IABP — distal to take-off of left subclavian

CVP line — above right atrium

Swan-Ganz catheter — proximal pulmonary artery (right side more common)

Pacemaker — tip of right ventricle; need lateral, too.

Chest tube — medial to inner rib margin...

Figure C-47

On the portable AP chest x-ray, the proper location for a chest tube placed to drain pleural fluid is _____ to the _____ of the _____ .

medial
inner margin
ribs

The tip of the CVP line must be in an _____ to record accurately the central venous pressure. It should lie distal to the anterior _____ . Two common complications of CVP line insertion are _____ and _____ .

intrathoracic position

first rib

pneumothorax
pleural effusion

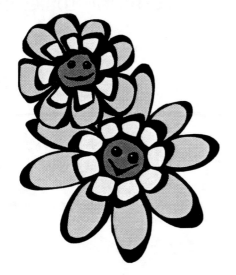

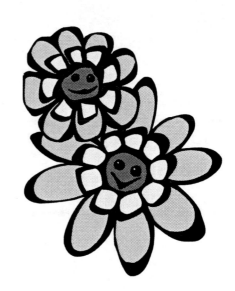

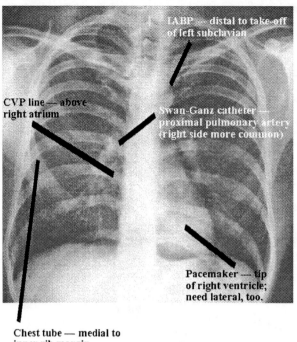

IABP — distal to take-off of left subclavian

CVP line — above right atrium

Swan-Ganz catheter — proximal pulmonary artery (right side more common)

Pacemaker — tip of right ventricle; need lateral, too.

Chest tube — medial to inner rib margin...

Figure C-47

In the unwedged position, the pulmonary artery catheter tip should be in the left or right _____ within _____ of the _____. If the tip is advanced too far, _____ of the lung may occur. If the tip migrates back into the right ventricle, _____ are possible.	central pulmonary artery 1-2 cm vertebral margin infarction ventricular arrhythmias

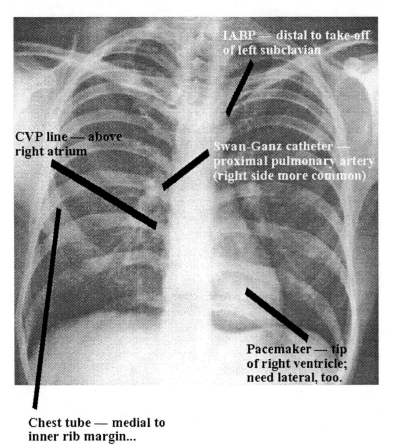

IABP — distal to take-off of left subclavian

CVP line — above right atrium

Swan-Ganz catheter — proximal pulmonary artery (right side more common)

Pacemaker — tip of right ventricle; need lateral, too.

Chest tube — medial to inner rib margin...

Figure C-47

The tip of an intra-aortic balloon pump (IABP) should lie just distal to the _____, roughly at the level of the _____. The balloon can be seen when it inflates during _____ as a _____ filling defect in the aorta.	left subclavian artery aortic knob diastole radiolucent

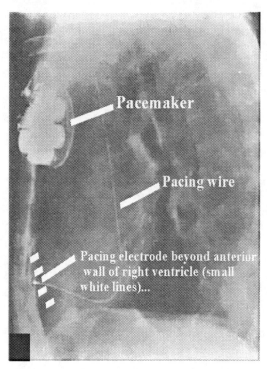

Permanent cardiac pacemaker

Figure C-49

| A ventricular pacing electrode should lie in the _____ of the _____ ventricle. On the AP film, the tip of the catheter should be just to the _____ of the vertebral margin. In the lateral film, the electrode tip should _____ towards the _____ of the ——— ventricle. | apex
right

left

curve
anterior border
right |

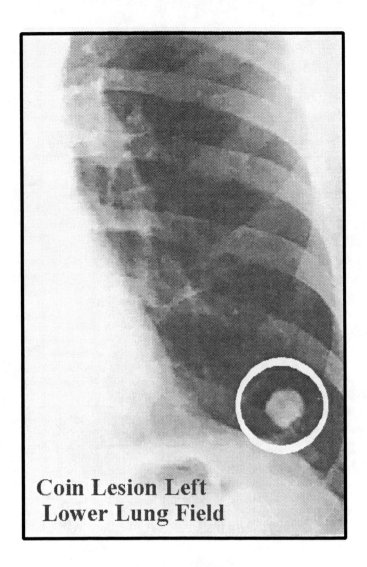

Coin Lesion Left
Lower Lung Field

Figure C-51

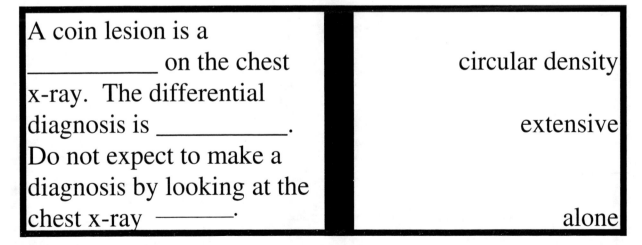

A coin lesion is a
_____ on the chest
x-ray. The differential
diagnosis is _____.
Do not expect to make a
diagnosis by looking at the
chest x-ray ———.

circular density

extensive

alone

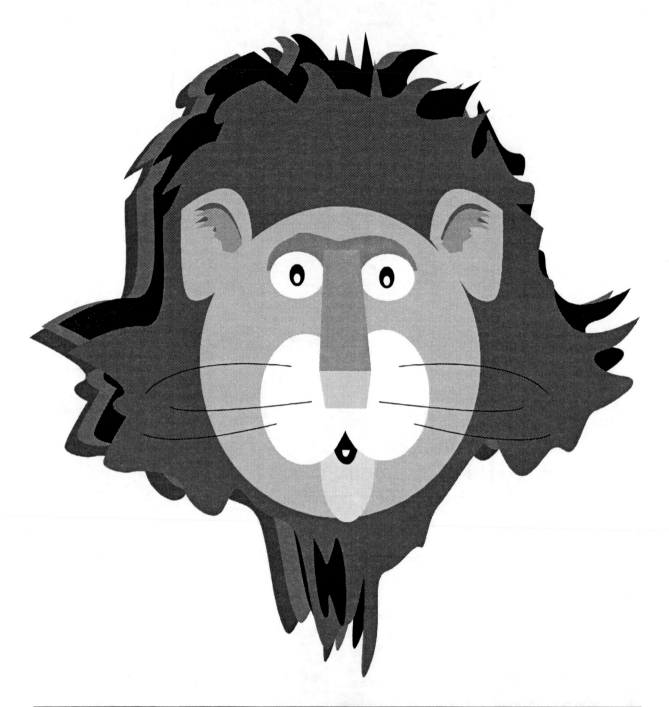

Patients with a life-threatening illness may still have a _____ chest x-ray.

normal

The Abdomen

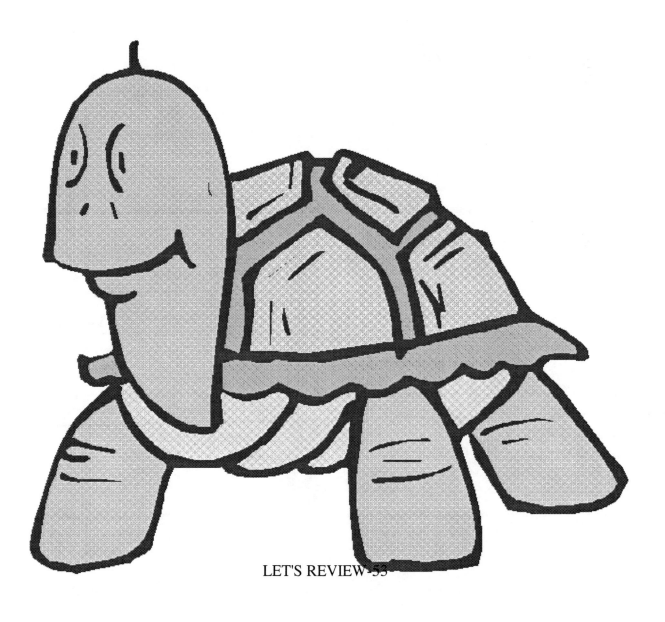

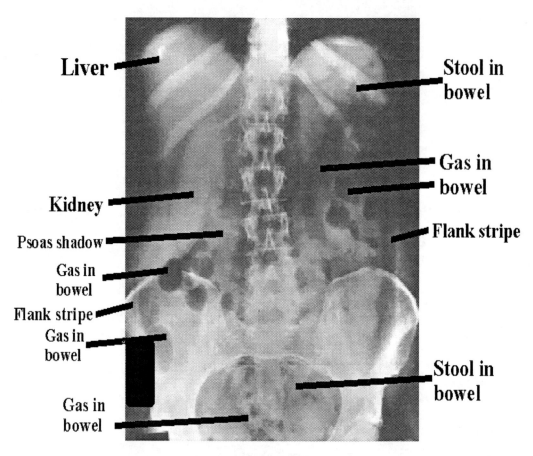

Liver

Stool in bowel

Gas in bowel

Kidney

Flank stripe

Psoas shadow

Gas in bowel

Flank stripe

Gas in bowel

Stool in bowel

Gas in bowel

Figure A-1

Think of the belly as a tree. The trunk of the tree is the _____, and the base is the _____. The tree trunk is "supported" on each side by the _____ while the lower ribs form the _____ of the tree.

vertebral column

upper pelvis

psoas muscle shadows

upper branches

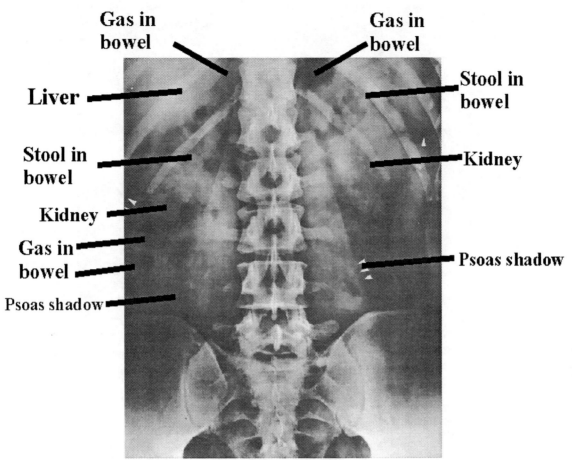

Gas in bowel

Gas in bowel

Liver

Stool in bowel

Stool in bowel

Kidney

Kidney

Gas in bowel

Psoas shadow

Psoas shadow

Figure A-2

The psoas shadows should be relatively _____. Otherwise, look for overlying _____ or intraperitoneal _____.	distinct stool fluid

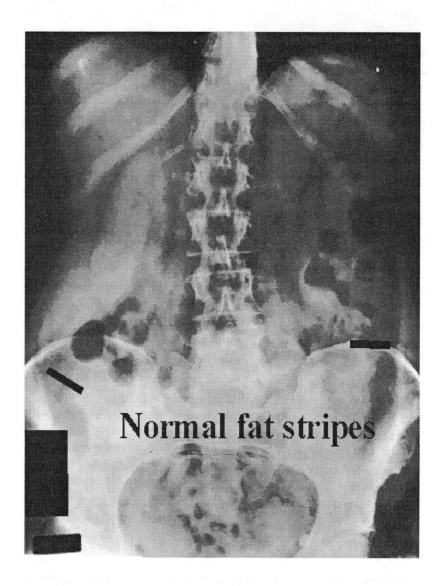

Normal fat stripes

Figure A-3

"Balloons" in the belly are usually _____!	abnormal
Just because you see stool in the abdomen doesn't mean the patient has _____.	constipation

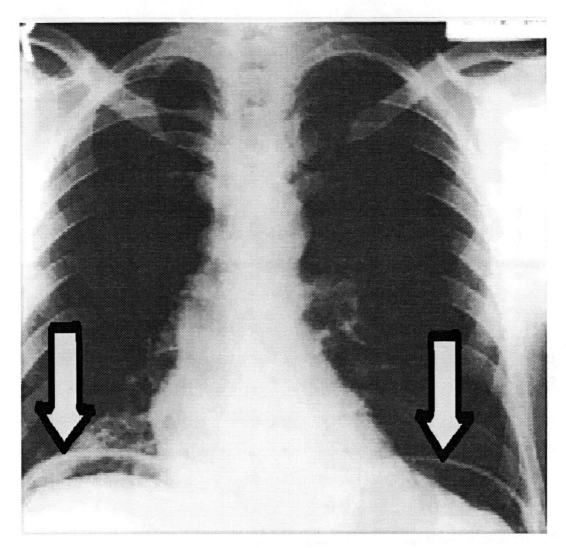

Bilateral "paper-thin" diaphragm indicating intraperitoneal free air...

Figure A-7

"The diaphragm should never be _____; if it is, there's _____ within... the _____!"	paper-thin free air peritoneum

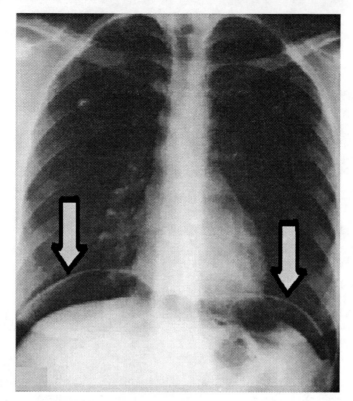

**"Paper-thin" diaphragms
due to free intraperitoneal air...**

Figure A-5

Free air is only visible in _____ of cases of documented hollow viscus rupture! If you strongly suspect the presence of rupture and don't see free air on the x-ray, try getting a _____ — very small amounts of intraperitoneal free air are seen as _____ in the belly.	85% noncontrast abdominal CT scan dark "spots"

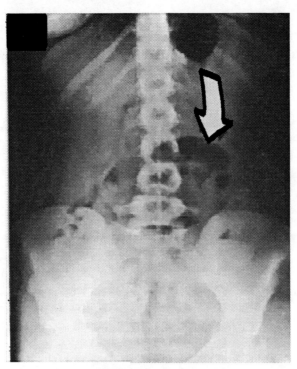

**"Bent-finger" sign indicating
localized ileus in small bowel...**

Figure A-9

Typically, you don't see small bowel on the normal film; if you do, it's limited to _____ that are _____ in width.	one or two small loops less than 2.5 cm
An isolated loop of dilated small bowel overlying an irritated viscus is often called a "_____" or "_____" and represents a _____ due to _____.	sentinel loop bent-finger sign localized ileus inflammation

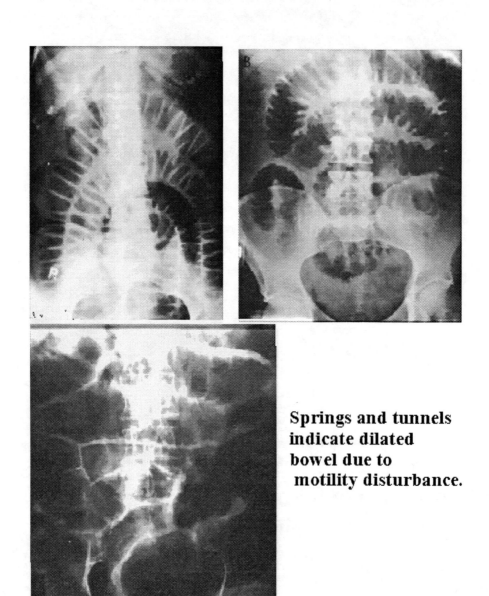

Springs and tunnels indicate dilated bowel due to motility disturbance.

Figure A-10

The "ST changes" of motility disturbance are _____ and _____.

springs
tunnels

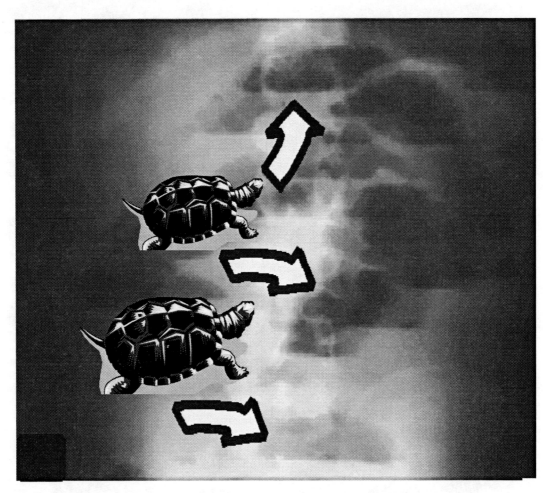

Note the close resemblance of air-fluid levels to the side view of a turtle's shell!

Figure A-12

Trapped fluid in dilated loops of bowel (air-fluid levels) look somewhat like _____.

turtle shells

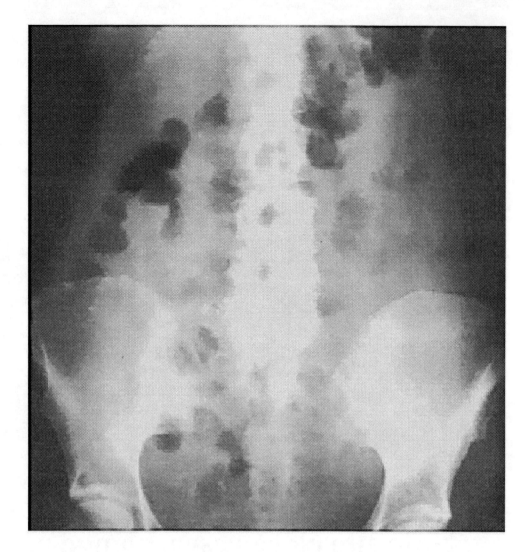

Diffuse abdominal haziness with obliteration of psoas shadows due to intraperitoneal fluid collection.

Figure A-13

Intraperitoneal fluid collection will blur out _____, which gives the abdomen a _____ appearance.	normal (psoas) shadows hazy

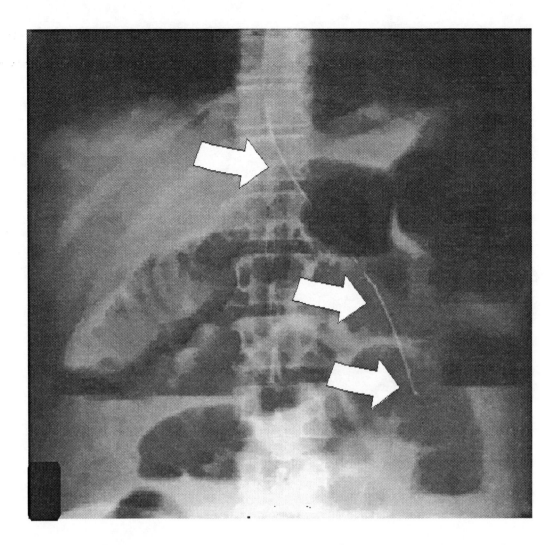

Normally positioned
nasogastric tube...

Figure A-15

The tip and side hole of a nasogastric tube should lie beyond the _____ and into the _____ on the AP film.	esophagogastric junction stomach

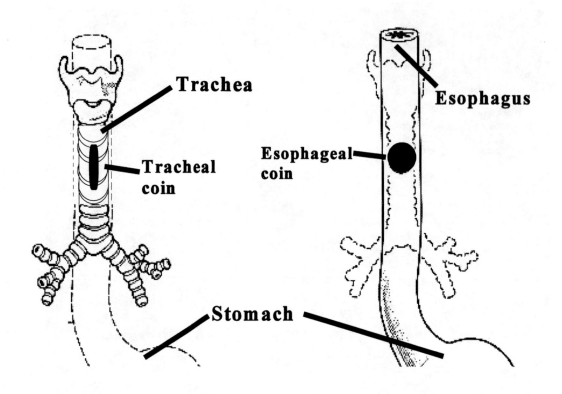

Figure A-16

When you see a radiopaque foreign body at the clavicle level that appears flat on the PA/AP chest film, strongly suspect it is in the _____.

esophagus

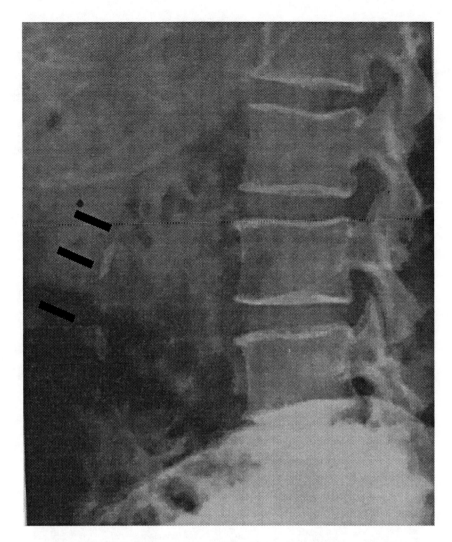

Calcification in anterior aorta suggests AAA!
Figure A-20

Eggshell calcification in the vicinity of the aorta is due to _____ until proven otherwise.	abdominal aortic aneurysm

BONES

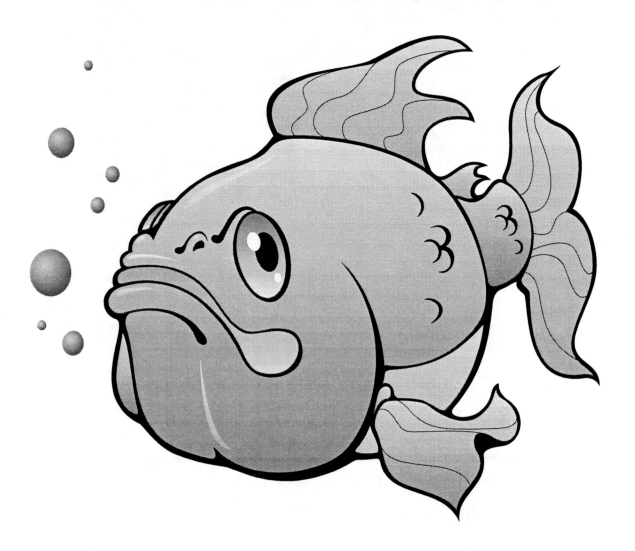

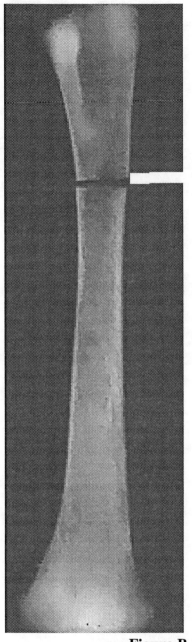

Fracture line...

Figure B-1

Bones are _____,
when they're _____,
they're _____.

smooth
not smooth
broken

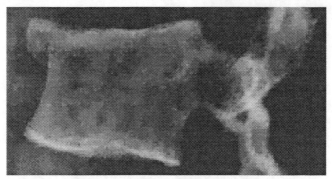

Vertebral compression fracture...

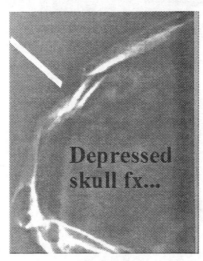

Depressed
skull fx...

Figure B-2

When bony fragments are impacted or compacted together (e.g., compression fracture, impacted hip fracture), the result is increased _____, more _____ to the passage of x-rays, and a "_____" at the point of bony overlap.	bony density resistance white line

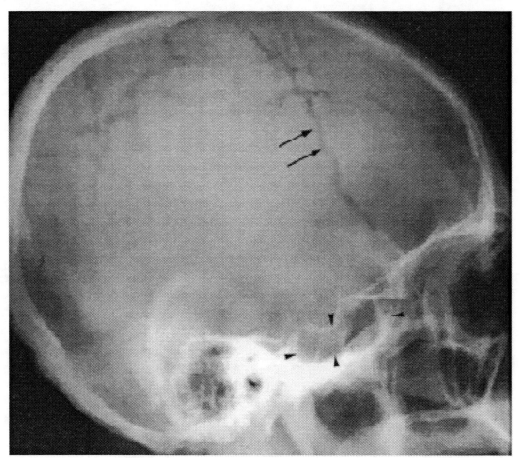

We're all scarecrows on a lateral skull film!

Figure B-4

None of us "have a _____" on the normal skull film.

brain

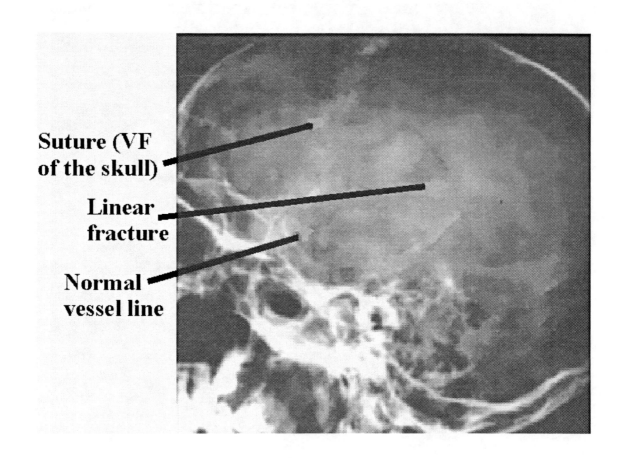

Suture (VF of the skull)

Linear fracture

Normal vessel line

Figure B-7

Suture lines form a unique saw-tooth pattern resembling _____. Thus, "v-fib of the skull" is almost always a _____.

ventricular fibrillation

suture line

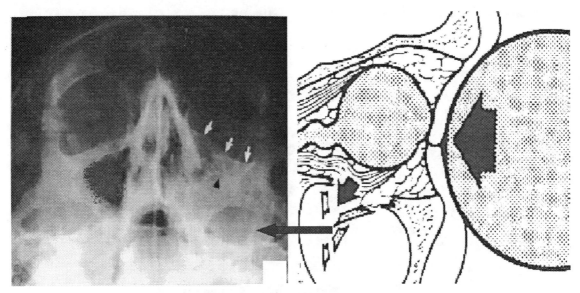

Orbital blow-out fracture leads to clouding of left maxillary sinus...

Figure B-8

In a blow-out fracture of the orbit, bone fragments and associated tissue are forced into the underlying _____. Despite the highest quality orbital films, seeing the fracture line itself is often _____.

maxillary sinus

difficult

The Vertebral Column, Its Sections and Curves

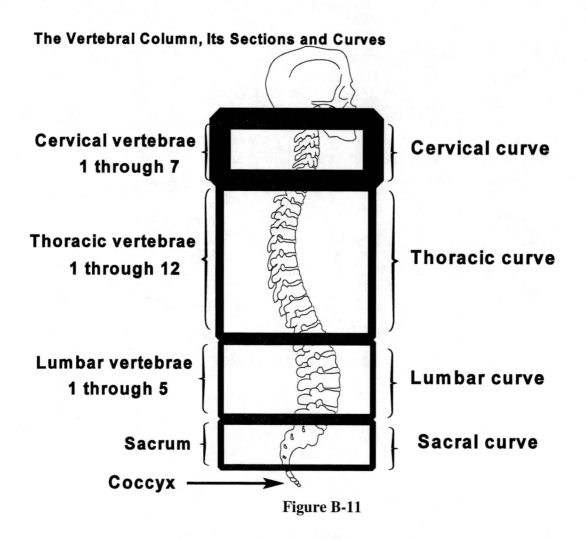

Cervical vertebrae 1 through 7 — Cervical curve

Thoracic vertebrae 1 through 12 — Thoracic curve

Lumbar vertebrae 1 through 5 — Lumbar curve

Sacrum — Sacral curve

Coccyx ⟶

Figure B-11

The most frequently injured area of the spine is the _____, followed by the _____. The thoracic spine is rarely injured with the exception of relatively minor _____.

lumbosacral spine
cervical spine

compression fractures

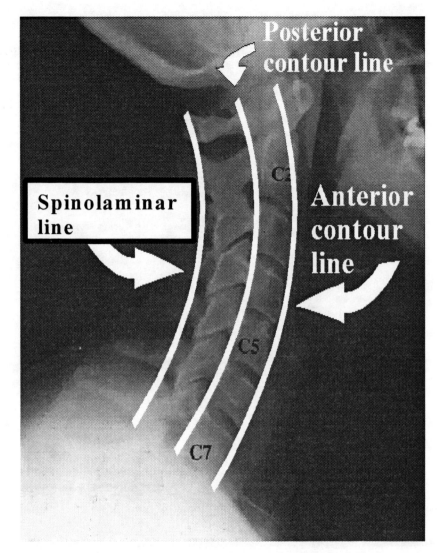

Posterior
contour line

Spinolaminar
line

C2

Anterior
contour
line

C5

C7

The three normal lines
of contour in the C-spine...

Figure B-16

When viewing a lateral spine film, ask yourself "Do we _____?"	line up

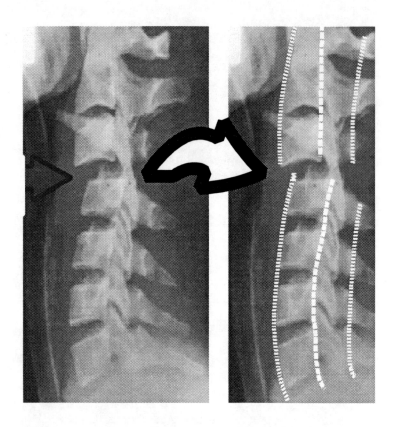

We DON'T line up!

Figure B-18

Regardless which portion of the spine, if the front and back of the vertebral bodies don't _____, assume the patient has an unstable spine with a potential risk of injury to the _____.

line up

spinal cord

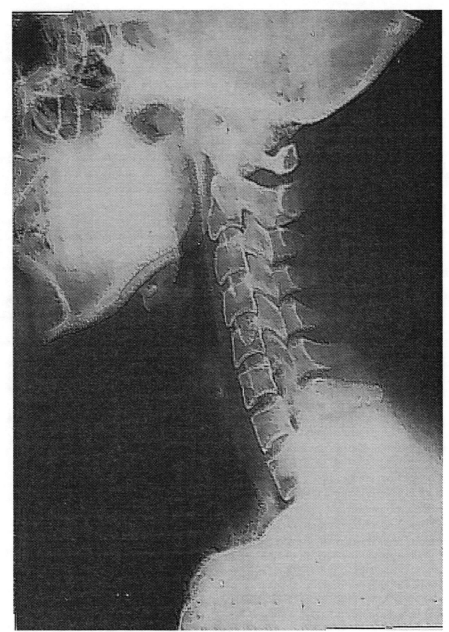

Figure B-17 — Normal Lateral Neck

Follow each vertebra from anterior to posterior to avoid missing a_____ injury.

posterior element

Normal vs Compression Fx

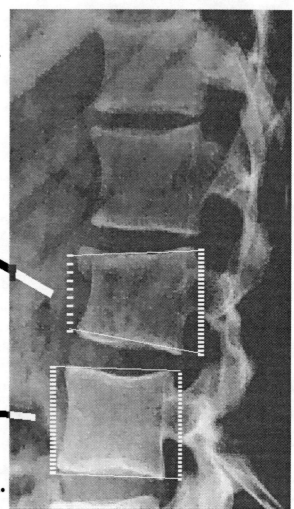

Vertebral compression fracture; anterior (front) height less than posterior (back) height; shaped like a trapezoid.

Normal square to rectangular-shaped vertebral body; front and back heights equal.

Figure B-23

Vertebral compression fractures typically result in a _____ vertebral body, with the _____ significantly (> 1-2 mm) less than the _____.	trapezoidal shaped anterior height posterior height

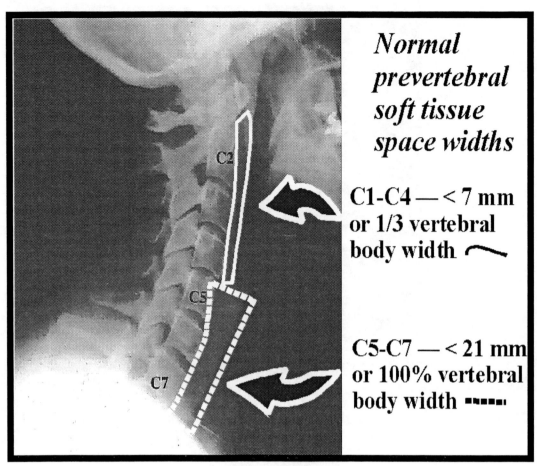

Figure B-19

The prevertebral space from C1 - C4 should be no wider than _____ or _____; below the larynx, from C5 - C7, the normal space is wider — no greater than _____ or _____.

7 mm
one-third the width of the vertebral body

21 mm
100% of the width of the vertebral body

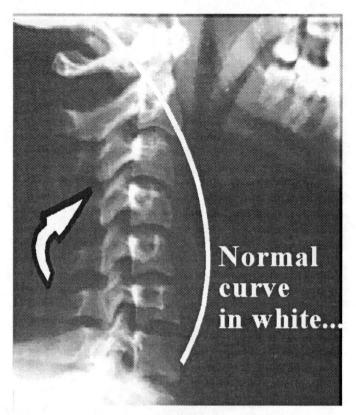

**Reversal of the normal cervical curve —
no fx seen; film ABNORMAL!!**

Figure B-21

Subtle signs of C-spine fractures include _____ in the prevertebral space, _____, and _____ or _____ of the normal _____.	soft tissue swelling loose bodies straightening reversal curve

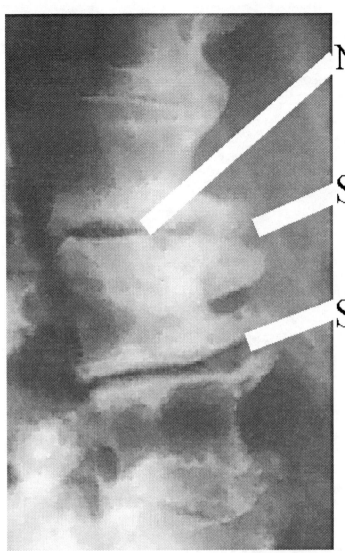

Narrowing

Severe lipping

Spurs, fusion

Figure B-14

Anywhere from 50 - 85% of persons without any symptoms have abnormal _____ spine x-rays, most commonly showing _____.

lumbosacral

degenerative changes

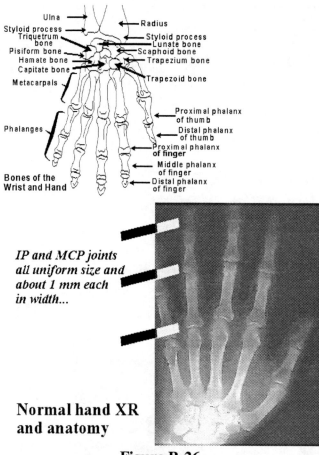

Ulna
Styloid process
Triquetrum bone
Pisiform bone
Hamate bone
Capitate bone
Metacarpals

Radius
Styloid process
Lunate bone
Scaphoid bone
Trapezium bone
Trapezoid bone

Phalanges

Proximal phalanx of thumb
Distal phalanx of thumb
Proximal phalanx of finger
Middle phalanx of finger

Bones of the Wrist and Hand

Distal phalanx of finger

IP and MCP joints all uniform size and about 1 mm each in width...

Normal hand XR and anatomy

Figure B-26

The spaces at the interphalangeal (IP) and metacarpal-phalangeal (MCP) joints should be _____ and about _____ each. Narrowing of this space on the AP view may indicate a severe _____, best seen on a _____ view.	uniform (equal) one mm misalignment lateral

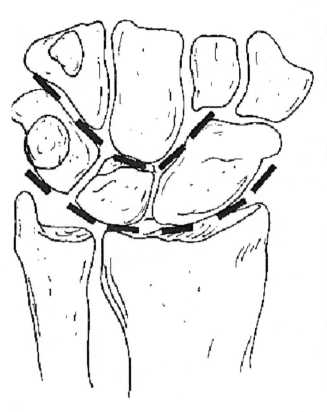 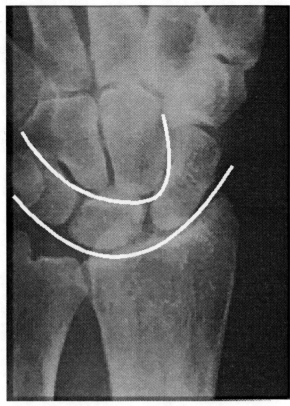

Normal lines of carpal alignment on AP view...

Figure B-29

There is no such thing as a "sprained wrist" until you completely rule out a _____ fracture.

navicular (scaphoid)

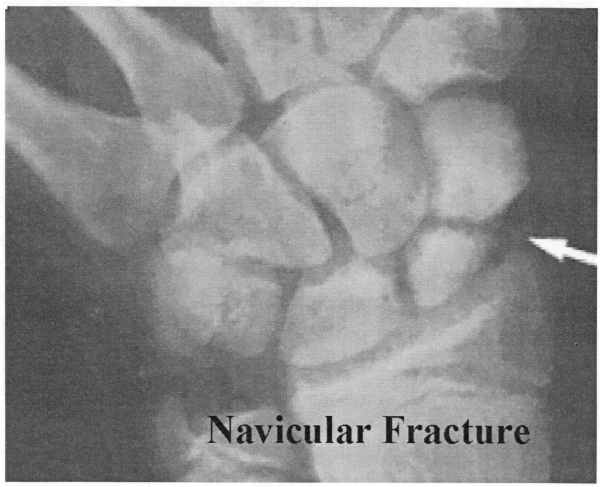

Figure B-32

The most commonly fractured bone in the wrist is the _____ or _____; the most commonly dislocated bone in the wrist is the _____.

navicular
scaphoid bone

lunate bone

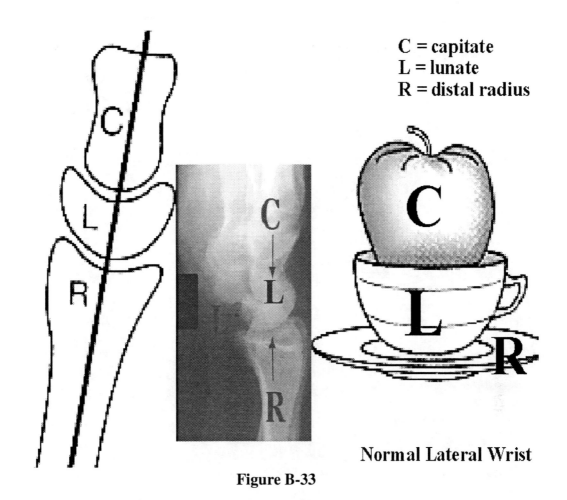

C = capitate
L = lunate
R = distal radius

Normal Lateral Wrist

Figure B-33

On the lateral wrist film, the outlines of the distal radius, lunate, and capitate form a series of shadows that resembles a _____ (distal radius) with a _____ sitting on top of it (lunate) and an _____ sitting in the cup (capitate).	saucer cup apple

Lunate Dislocation (anterior)

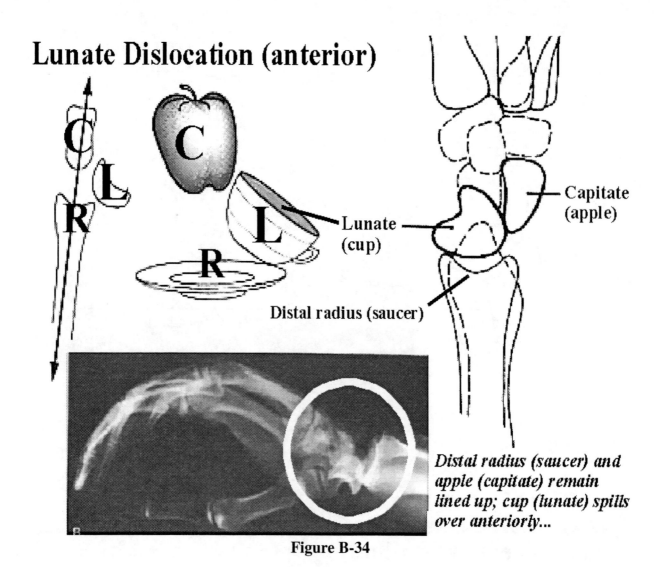

Capitate (apple)

Lunate (cup)

Distal radius (saucer)

Distal radius (saucer) and apple (capitate) remain lined up; cup (lunate) spills over anteriorly...

Figure B-34

Regarding the lateral wrist film: "You should never see the _____ in the wrist; if you do, there's a _____ twist!"

moon

lunate bone

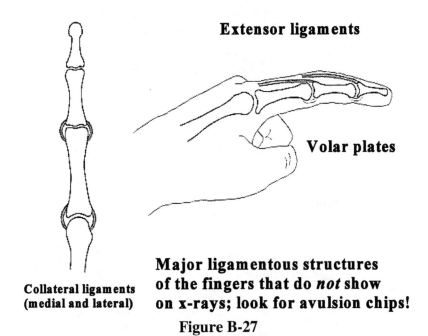

Extensor ligaments

Volar plates

**Collateral ligaments
(medial and lateral)**

**Major ligamentous structures
of the fingers that do *not* show
on x-rays; look for avulsion chips!**

Figure B-27

There are three soft tissue structures in the fingers that are at high risk for injury — _____, _____, and _____.

extensor tendons
volar plates
collateral tendons

_____ are small, round bones located within tendons and sometimes mistaken for fracture fragments. The largest of these in the body is the _____.

Sesamoid bones

patella

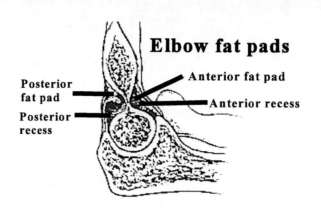

Elbow fat pads

Posterior fat pad

Anterior fat pad

Anterior recess

Posterior recess

(Posterior normally not seen)

(Anterior normally visible)

Abnormal = anterior FP "sailed forward" *or* posterior FP visible at all...

(Suggests joint effusion)

Normal

Abnormal

Figure B-38

An _____ fat pad flat against the elbow joint is normal; if it's "_____," it's always abnormal. A visible posterior fat pad is also always _____. These abnormal findings indicate the presence of _____ — a common finding with occult fracture of the _____.

anterior

sailed out

abnormal

effusion in the joint

radial head

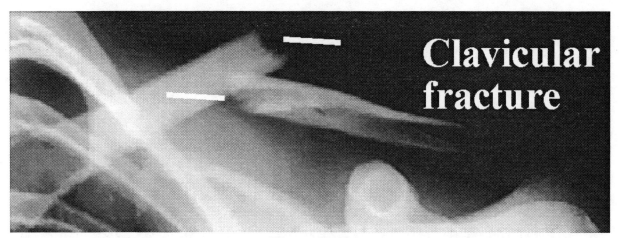

Figure B-42

Life-threatening complications from clavicle fractures include _____ and damage to _____.

pneumothorax
underlying vessels

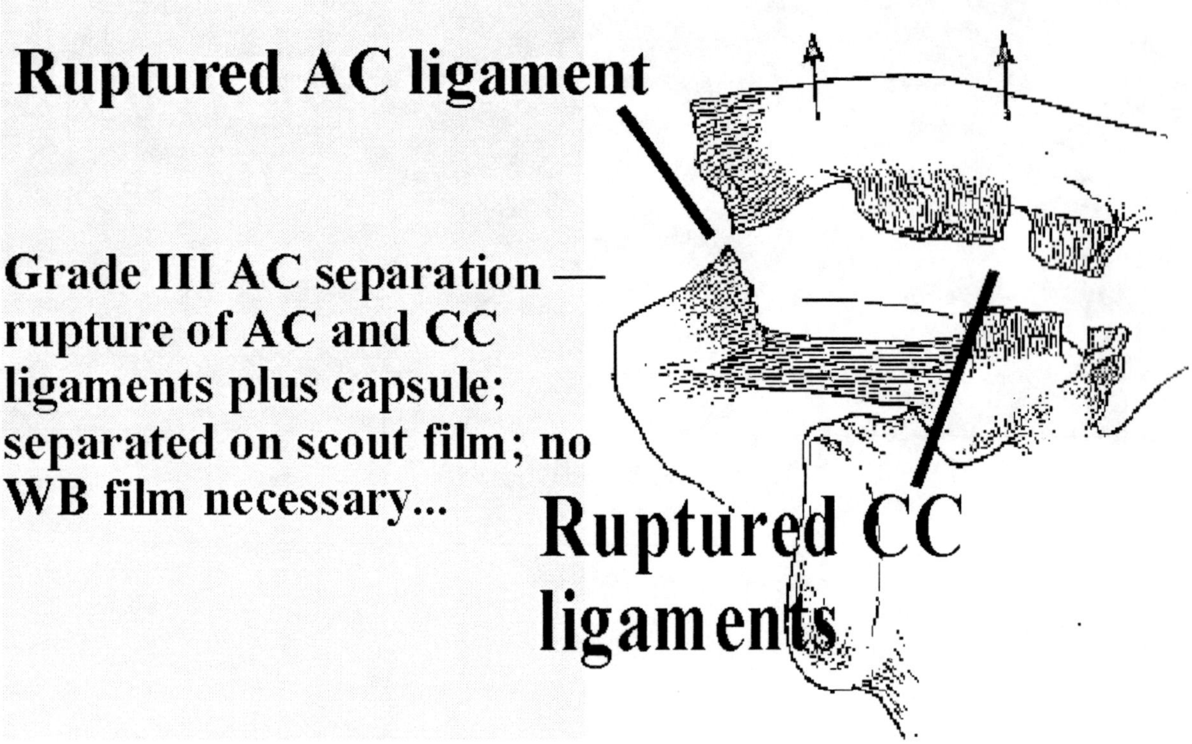

Ruptured AC ligament

Grade III AC separation — rupture of AC and CC ligaments plus capsule; separated on scout film; no WB film necessary...

Ruptured CC ligaments

Figure B-45

In a Grade III AC separation, there is _____ without any weight bearing. In a Grade I separation there is _____ with weight bearing. And, in a Grade II separation, there is _____ only during weight bearing.	complete separation no separation some separation

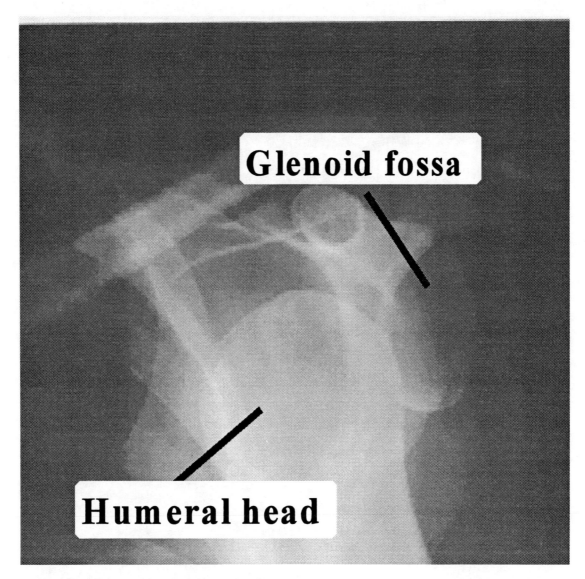

Glenoid fossa

Humeral head

Anterior dislocation — "The humerus doesn't live here anymore!"

Figure B-48

The most common shoulder dislocation is _____.	anterior

Overlap of humeral head on glenoid fossa...

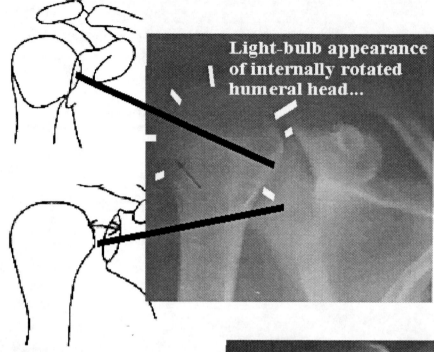

Light-bulb appearance of internally rotated humeral head...

Widening of joint space due to internal rotation...

(Note slightly asymmetrical "walking stick" appearance of normal humeral head...)

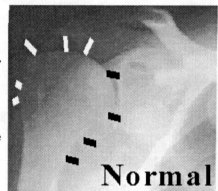

Normal

Figure B-49

Look for widening of the humeral-glenoid space as a sign of internal rotation and _____.

posterior dislocation

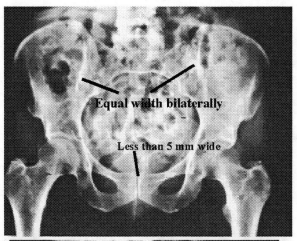

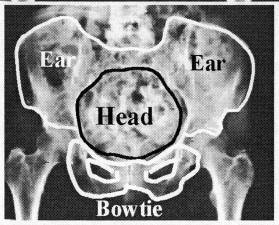

Normal Pelvis X-Ray

Figure B-50

On the normal pelvis film, the sacroiliac joint width should be _____ on both sides. The pubic symphysis should be no wider than _____ and the bones should be _____.	equal 5 mm smooth

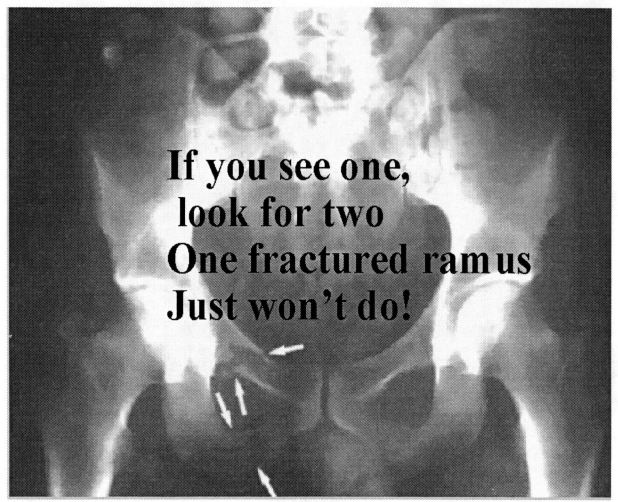

Figure B-51

Think of the pelvis as a _____; remember if one side of the "bow-tie" is broken, look for a fracture on the _____.

well-dressed animal

opposite side

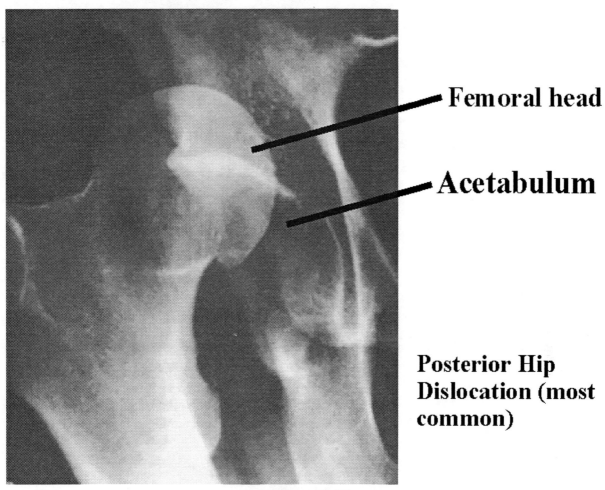

Femoral head

Acetabulum

Posterior Hip Dislocation (most common)

Figure B-55

The most common hip dislocation is _____.

posterior

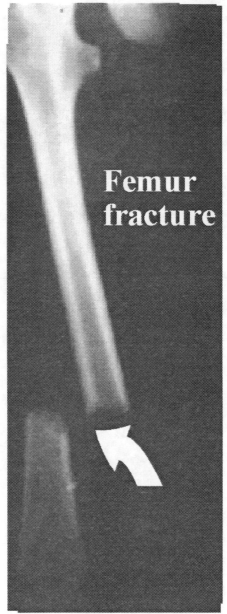

Figure B-57

Assume any patient with a femoral shaft fracture has lost at least _____ units of blood *per fracture* into the thigh.	two or three

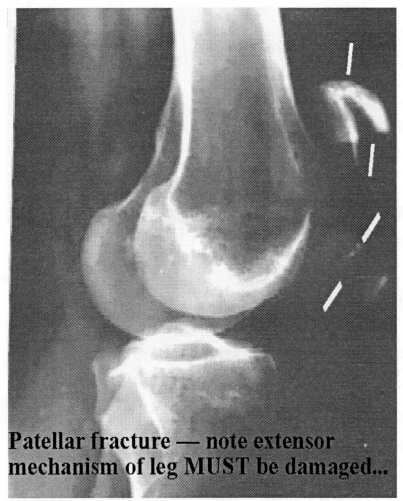

Patellar fracture — note extensor mechanism of leg MUST be damaged...

Figure B-60

Assume that any patient with a comminuted fracture of the patella also has significant damage to the _____.

Extensor mechanism of the knee

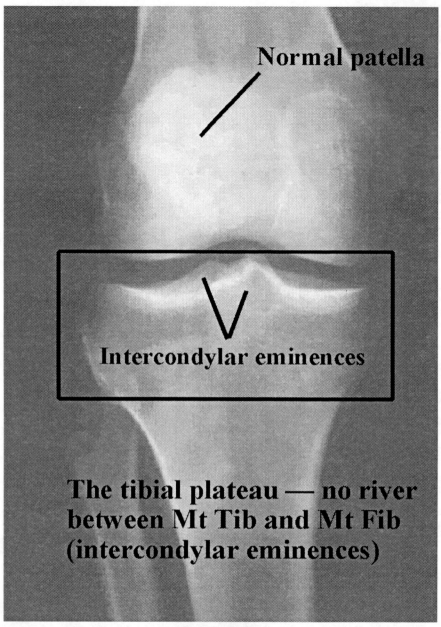

Normal patella

Intercondylar eminences

The tibial plateau — no river between Mt Tib and Mt Fib (intercondylar eminences)

Figure B-61

There should never be a _____ between "Mount Tib and Mount Fib." If so, within a ———— lives!

river

fracture

Peroneus brevis tendon avulsion

Peroneus brevis tendon

Peroneus brevis muscle

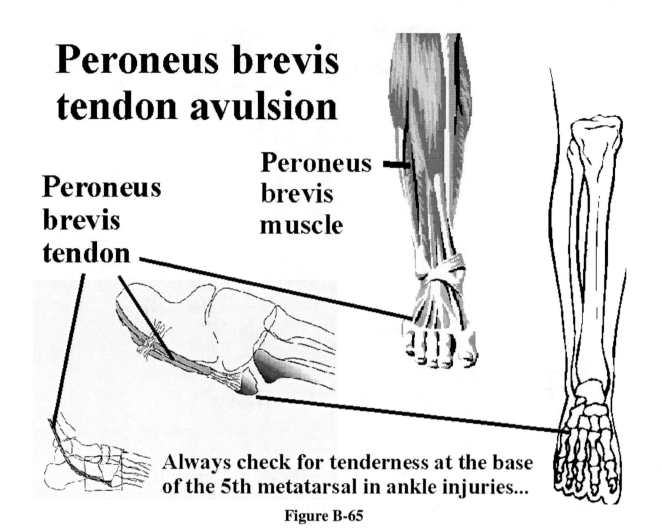

Always check for tenderness at the base of the 5th metatarsal in ankle injuries...

Figure B-65

In a patient with an ankle sprain, always check for _____ (fracture of the proximal fibula) and _____ (avulsion of peroneus brevis tendon).	calf tenderness tenderness at the base of the 5th toe

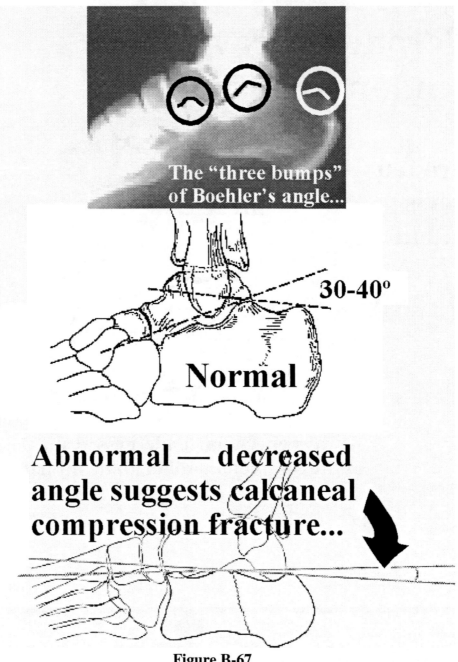

The "three bumps"
of Boehler's angle...

30-40°

Normal

Abnormal — decreased angle suggests calcaneal compression fracture...

Figure B-67

Most calcaneal fractures are caused by _____ — look for _____.

falls
associated injuries

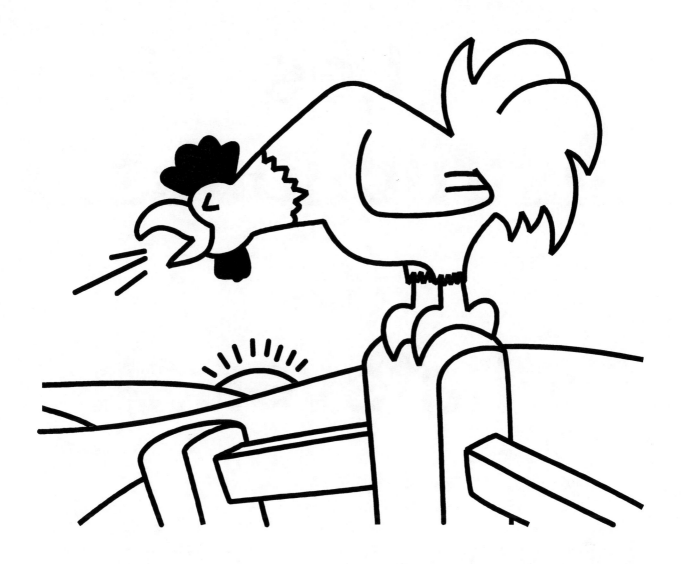

Now, let's try some unknowns...

Les instructiones... (or whatever...):

Look at the film while covering the answer in the right-hand column. <u>After</u> you've formed an opinion about the film, compare your reading with the answer. If we disagree, make sure (please!!) that you understand why...

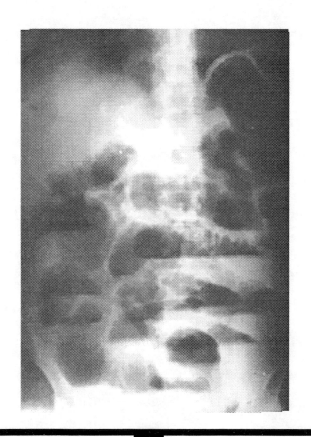

35 year old male with nausea, vomiting, and abdominal pain for three days.

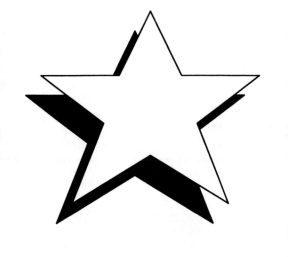

I see multiple "turtle shells," indicating a motility disturbance, for any of a number of reasons. Remember the "shells" indicate air fluid levels in dilated bowel. Without additional clinical information, it is *impossible* to reach further conclusions from this film...

45 year old female with a history of rheumatoid arthritis who complains of spontaneous pain and swelling in her elbow. The prepatellar bursa is swollen and red. There is a small abrasion over her posterior olecranon area.

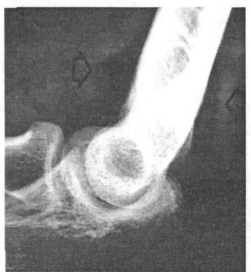

There are abnormal anterior and posterior fat pad signs, indicating joint effusion. There is no history of trauma, so the effusion might be due to rheumatoid arthritis. On the other hand, could she have septic arthritis *and* septic bursitis — what about that little scrape on her elbow? In the presence of clinical septic bursitis, a positive fat pad sign strongly suggests joint space infection as well.

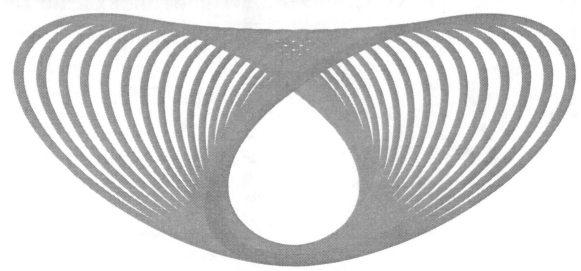

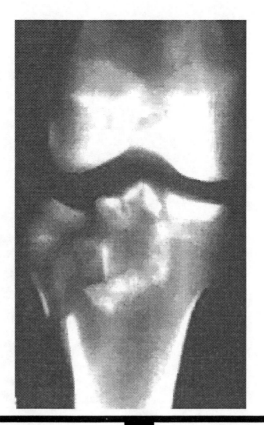

56 year old male who limped into your clinic complaining of knee pain. He also appeared to be intoxicated.

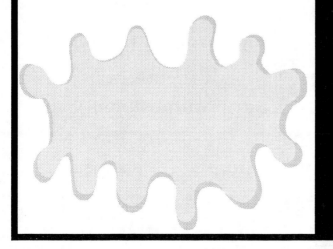

So much for the (incorrect) "maxim" that people don't walk on broken legs... The tibial plateau fracture fragment is laterally and inferiorly displaced. Note the "river" between the intercondylar eminences ("Mount Tib" and "Mount Fib") indicating the fracture line.

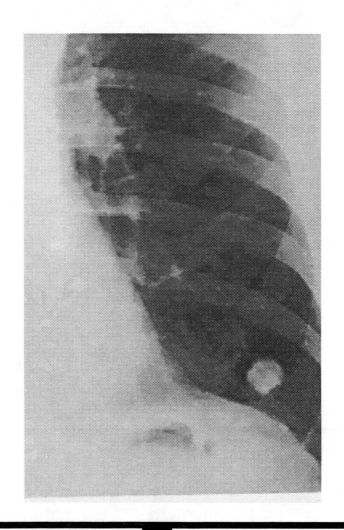

Healthy 36 year old male, nonsmoker, who had this chest film done during a routine pre-employment exam.

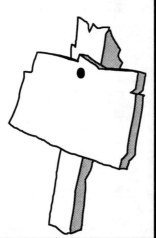

Assuming what we *don't see* is o.k. (otherwise symmetrical with markings all the way out), the patient has a 1-2 cm round density in the left lower lung field. Potential causes range from TB to tumor to calcified foreign body...

70 year old female with a history of breast cancer; she leaned on her right arm and developed sudden and severe pain.

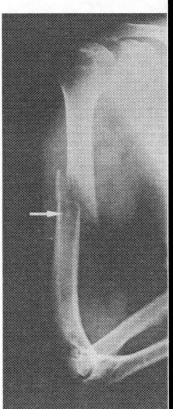

Bones are smooth; when they're not smooth, they're broken. Did you note the radiolucent area of bone below the fracture line? Scattered decreases in bone density ("color") are usually bad news. Though we can't prove it with the film alone, a pathologic fracture through an area of metastatic tumor to the humerus seems very likely.

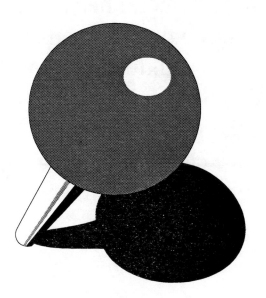

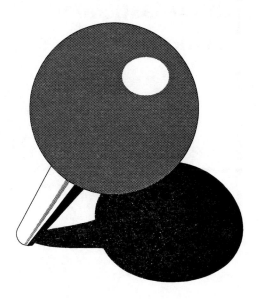

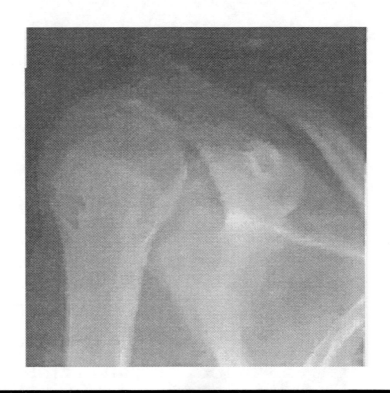

25 year old male who complained of sudden right shoulder pain and inability to move his arm after a particularly enthusiastic football tackle.

Without a comparison view, this posterior shoulder dislocation may be difficult to see. Note the abnormal symmetry of the humeral head (like a "lightbulb," instead of like a "walking stick.") Also note the widening of the glenohumeral space cause by internal rotation of the humeral head.

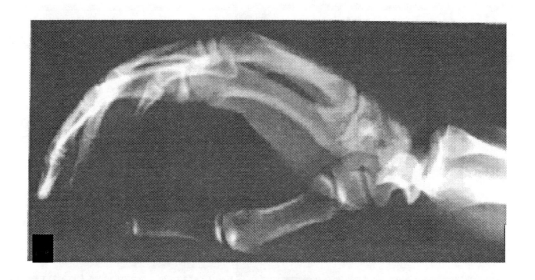

22 year old female who slipped on an icy sidewalk. She complains of palmar wrist tenderness and is unable to move her hand at the wrist joint.

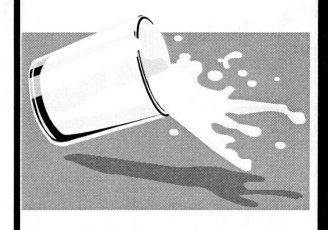

You immediately notice the "moon in the wrist," indicating a "lunate bone twist!" The normal linear orientation of the distal radius ("saucer"), lunate ("cup"), and capitate ("apple") is disrupted by anterior (palmar) dislocation of the lunate. The radius ("saucer") and capitate ("apple") remain aligned while the "cup" (lunate) "spills over." This represents a lunate dislocation.

28 year old male with weakness, weight loss, and night sweats over the past two months.

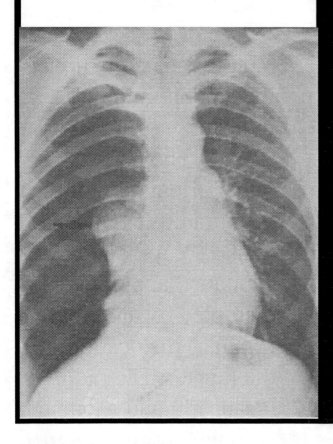

Though the lung markings go all the way out, there is significant asymmetry at the right hilum. The cause is a radiopaque density which obliterates the right heart border. The remainder of the lung fields are o.k. Potential causes for this "mass" are numerous and include: sarcoidosis, bronchogenic carcinoma, TB, pneumonia, pulmonary cyst, pleural tumor... In other words, the film by itself indicates the *finding* of a right hilar mass, *not* any particular diagnosis!

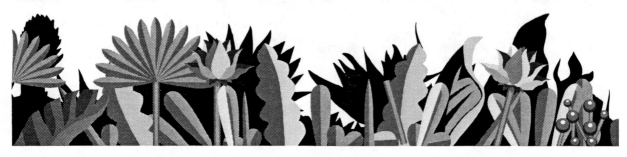

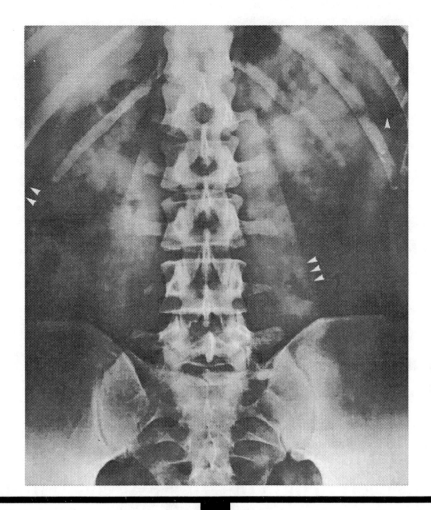

16 year old male with two days of periumbilical pain, now localized in the right lower quadrant. He has a fever, elevated WBC, and RLQ rebound tenderness. His appetite is markedly decreased.

Hope you realized that this patient presented with a "textbook" profile of appendicitis... at least this better be your first diagnostic consideration. The film, by the way, is completely normal! Remember, "a normal film does *not* mean a normal patient."

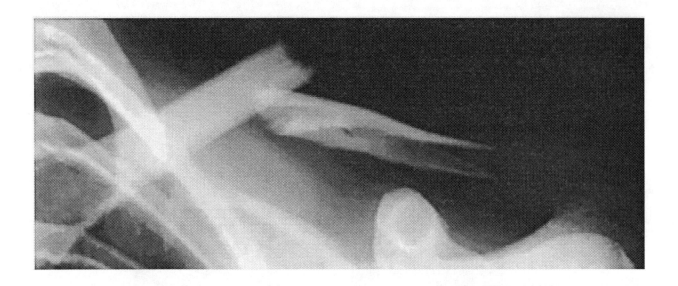

42 year old female falls at home against a set of drawers. She complains of severe "shoulder pain," and inability to move her left arm. On exam, she is only tender over her midclavicle.

The clavicular fracture is easy to see... Note that this film does *not*, however, allow us to rule out more severe potential associated injuries — such as underlying pneumothorax or subclavian vessel tear.

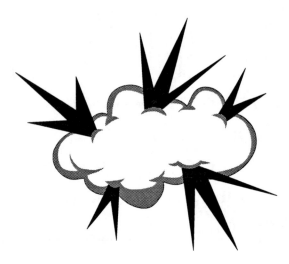
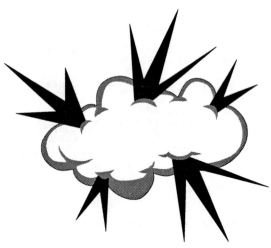

45 year old male smoker with shortness of breath and decreased exercise capacity over the past 2 months.

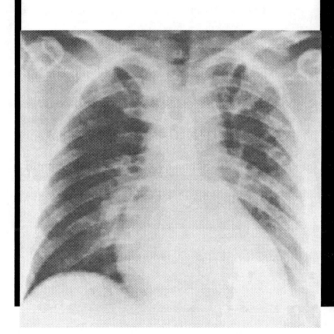

We're not symmetrical... there is blunting of the left costophrenic angle, suggesting pleural effusion. Remember — to blunt the angle, the posterior sulcus has to fill up first. So even minimal blunting suggests at least 250-500 cc of pleural fluid. As to the contents of the fluid — your guess is as good as mine without additional information... What other films might you obtain to confirm that the blunting is due to pleural fluid?

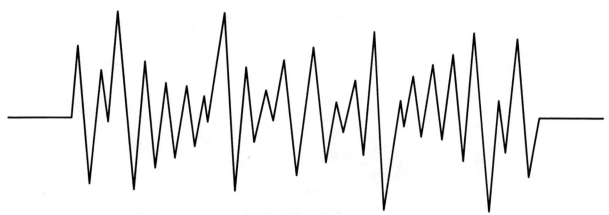

21 year old female with severe sore throat. She's unable to swallow and is drooling.

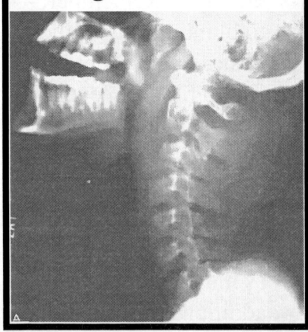

DANGER!! Note the marked prevertebral swelling in the upper cervical area. This suggests accumulation of fluid in the soft tissues. In trauma, this finding is due to occult spinal fracture until proven otherwise. In this case, a good possibility, especially in light of the clinical history, would be a retropharyngeal abscess.

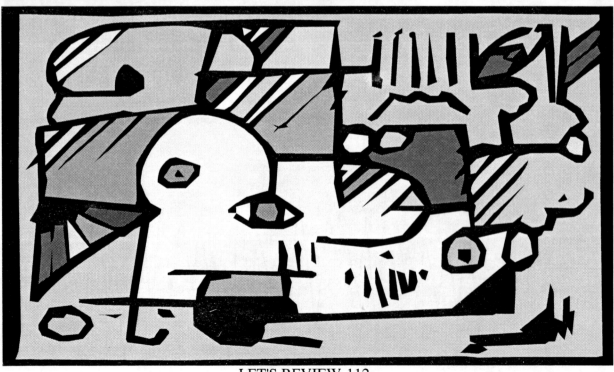

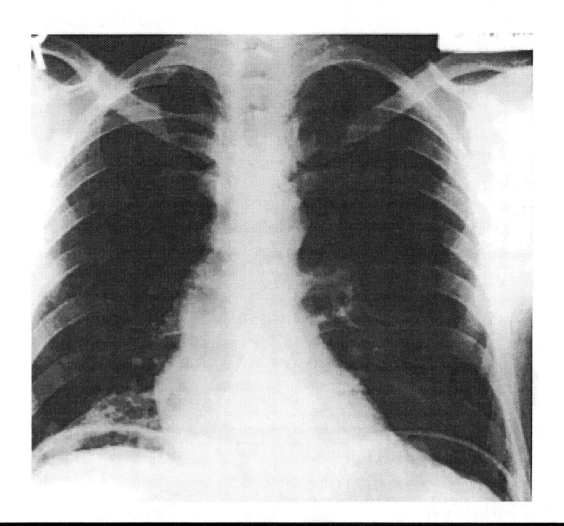

60 year old female with sudden onset of severe, midepigastric pain. Her abdomen is rigid on examination and no bowel sounds are present...

The diaphragm shadows should never be paper thin... if they are, there's free air within... the peritoneum! The finding of free air is often, though not always, due to ruptured hollow viscus (such as a peptic ulcer).

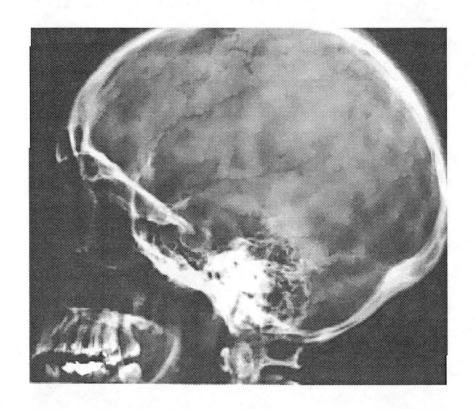

26 year old male involved in an altercation and hit in the head with a baseball bat. He was unconscious for about three minutes. Other than a strong odor of ethanol, his exam is now normal.

"We're all scarecrows on the lateral skull film!" No one has a brain — including health care providers who think that a "normal" skull film *really does* rule out intracranial injury. Especially with a period of unconsciousness for more than a few seconds, many consider a CT scan essential.

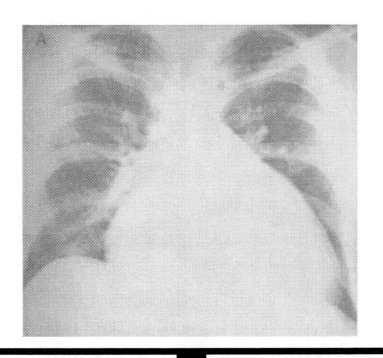

53 year old male with shortness of breath, worse when lying down, for the past four days...

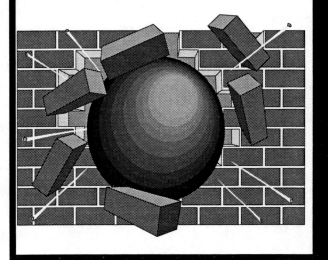

I bet your first tendency is to say "enlarged cardiac silhouette..." Mine was, too, until I looked at the ribs. This film represents an *inadequate* inspiratory effort — normally you should see at least 8-10 ribs. Since it's such a poor inspiration, the cardiac shadow is artificially magnified and the lung fields appear denser (whiter) than usual.

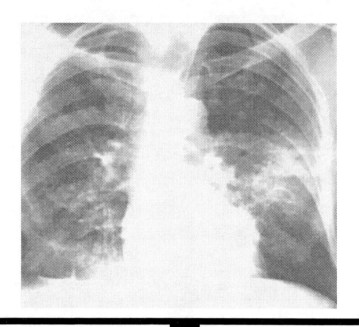

17 year old female with a productive cough, fever, and malaise for two days.

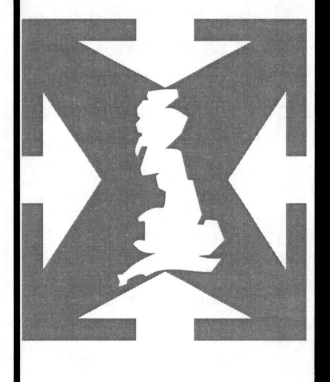

Asymmetrically abnormal! There are bilateral infiltrates. Both are patchy and probably involve the lower lobes (note sparing of heart border on left, and blurring of the medial diaphragm on the right). The cause is likely infectious, based on clinical information, but this infiltrate pattern, *by itself*, could be due to any collection of fluid within the lung parenchyma.

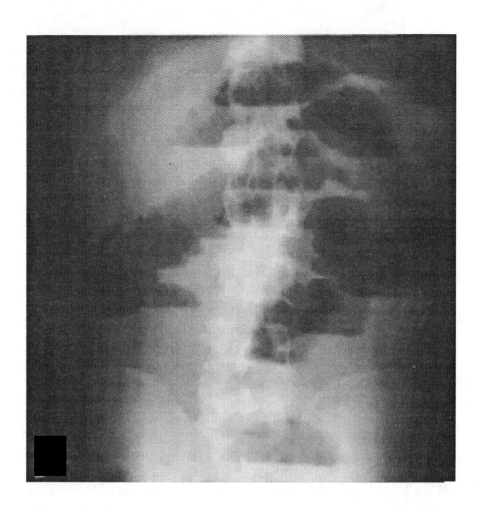

56 year old male with progressive abdominal distension, nausea, and vomiting.

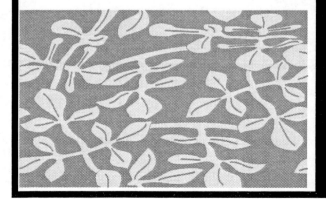

I see some "springs" in the right upper quadrant as well as several "turtle shells." These indicate dilated bowel and air-fluid levels — motility disturbance. We need further information to determine the actual cause...

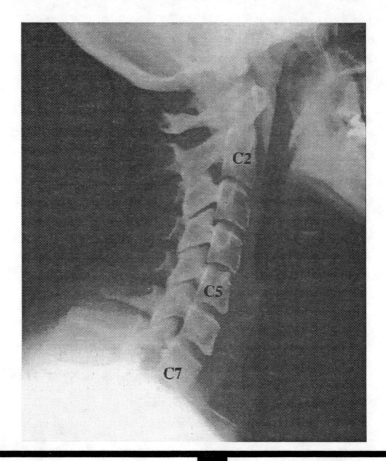

C2

C5

C7

19 year old male injured while playing football. He complains of severe posterior neck tenderness. The neurological examination is normal.

Remember — "a normal x-ray does *not* mean a normal patient." This film is quite normal... or is it? Look at the prevertebral tissues. There is significant swelling, especially anterior to C5. I'd get further films and consider a neck CT before ruling out a spine injury.

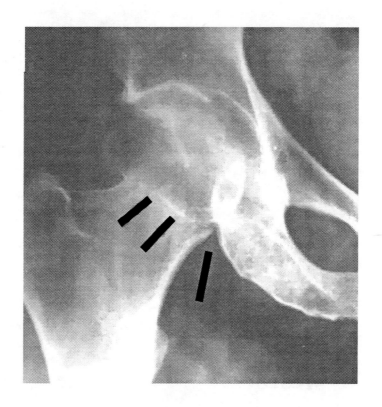

75 year old female who fell while trying to pick something up from the floor. She complains of severe right hip pain. Her right leg appears shortened and externally rotated.

Though the arrows make the sclerotic fracture line difficult to miss, a comparison view would have been most helpful. Also note the break in the cortex medially, near the pubic ramus. The white line forms as a result of trabecular bone being impacted (crushed) together.

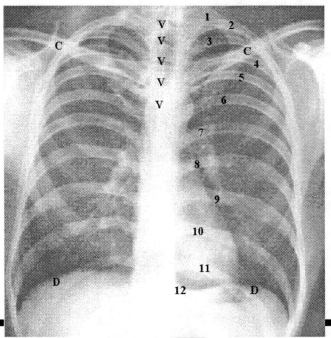

21 year old male who presents with severe shortness of breath, mild dry cough, and a room air pO_2 of 40 mm Hg (abnormally low).

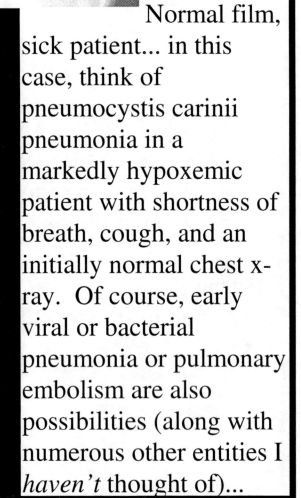

Normal film, sick patient... in this case, think of pneumocystis carinii pneumonia in a markedly hypoxemic patient with shortness of breath, cough, and an initially normal chest x-ray. Of course, early viral or bacterial pneumonia or pulmonary embolism are also possibilities (along with numerous other entities I *haven't* thought of)...

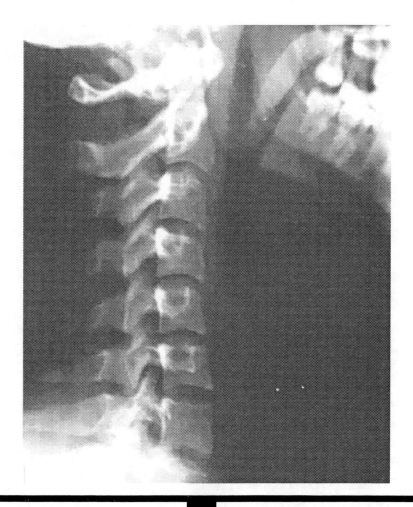

25 year old female who fell down a flight of stairs while intoxicated. Neurological exam is normal. She complains of severe posterior neck pain on exam.

This lady has straightening of the normal curve of the C-spine, suggesting muscle spasm secondary to an occult fracture. Though the bones sure look smooth to me, I'd immobilize her, obtain a neck CT, and consider consultation...

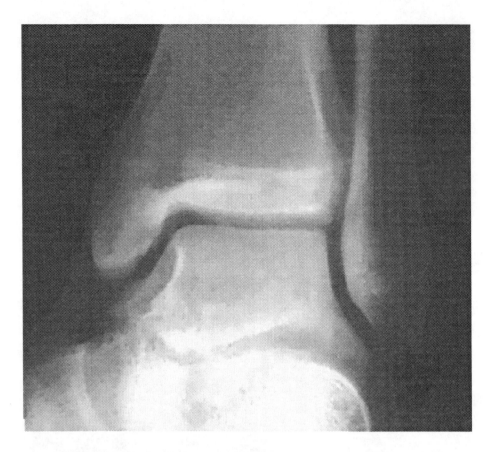

42 year old female who "twisted her ankle" while jogging. She is unable to bear any weight.

As is the case with many ankle injuries, the x-ray is normal while the ankle is not! Clinical exam in this particular patient revealed joint instability suggesting a very severe ligament tear *not* visible on the routine ankle series. Look at the patient, not just at the x-rays!

Now, I bet you <u>really</u> know this stuff...great job!

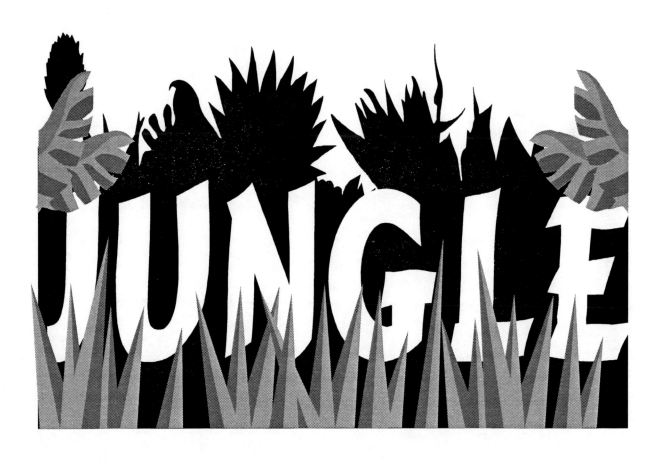

Section 5:

More Fun If You're Interested

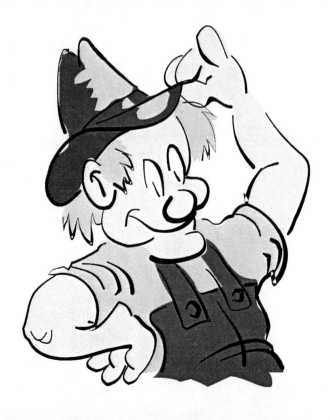

MORE FUN IF YOU'RE INTERESTED...

CONTENTS:

- Requisitions — How to order x-rays without getting a migraine...
- Patient preparation and care — My patients don't "code" in x-ray!
- Radiographic decision-making — Is there a method to our madness?
- X-ray triage — A great timesaver...
- Medical-legal aspects of x-rays — How to avoid the thrill of a summons and the agony of a deposition!

A Quick Note — the format of this section is somewhat different than the previous chapters. It's more of a summary outline. Where necessary, I've elaborated and provided references.

REQUISITIONS — HOW TO ORDER X-RAYS WITHOUT GETTING A MIGRAINE...

1. Bookkeeping information — name, hospital number, and patient's age. It's essential to have correct *identifying* information.

> *REMEMBER* — If you can't identify the patient, the film is worthless!

2. Purpose of the film — provide the radiographer with a brief indication of the reason for films. If the film is a "recheck," note the time interval since the last film. Also, note if a procedure has been done since the last

> *PLEASE* — Don't be *cute* and ask the radiologist to try and read the film without adequate clinical information. How would you like to read an EKG with only four leads, instead of twelve?

examination, such as thoracentesis, re-manipulation of a fracture, or passage of a catheter. State clinical information as:

- The chief medical complaint of the patient (for example, swelling, unexplained pain, limited range of motion, hemoptysis) or

- Rule out (R/O) fracture, foreign body, renal stone, pneumothorax, dissecting aortic aneurysm, cervical spine fractures...

3. The area to be examined — as a rule, rather than requesting particular views, designate the *area* to be examined. Be as specific as possible — this will permit the radiographer to take the most meaningful views of the indicated area, with the minimum radiation and expense to the patient. Take as few x-rays as possible.

> *REMEMBER* — **Work together with the radiographer as colleagues to determine the *best* views...**

PATIENT PREPARATION AND CARE — MY PATIENTS DON'T "CODE" IN X-RAY!

1. Who should go to the Radiology Department (x-ray department)? As a general rule, request portable films with *any* seriously compromised patient since the x-ray department is rarely equipped or staffed to handle a real crisis situation.

> *REMEMBER* — **A good radiographer can get a helpful portable film of just about any area of the body!**

2. Patient preparation before going to the x-ray department — disrobe the patient to the extent necessary to see what you need to; be certain that the area being filmed is totally clear of clothing or metal parts (including jewelry, safety pins in garments, and bra snaps), and clean.

3. How does the patient go to the x-ray department? Stretcher patients should travel to x-ray on stretchers, wheelchair patients in wheelchairs, and the rare walking patient accompanied by a health care professional. *Never* allow patients to wander off to x-ray and assume they will get there.

> *REMEMBER* — It's poor form when the patient takes an unplanned and unescorted tour of the Administrator's office...

Department policy should state that *all* patients be accompanied to the x-ray waiting area.

4. With whom? Don't allow any acutely ill (including head trauma) or unstable patients to wait in the hall unattended. *Do not* expect the x-ray department to watch the patient — the clinician *must* provide appropriate patient coverage. Remember that the busy radiology department cannot closely monitor a patient with head injury (or any other sick patient, for that matter), who is lying unattended in the waiting area. If not carefully

> *CLINICAL HINT* — Though some radiology departments have specially-trained staff to take care of sick patients, the responsibility *usually* lies with the clinician (*you*) who sent the patient to x-ray in the first place!

watched, a lethargic patient may rapidly become comatose before returning from x-ray without anyone's being aware of a deterioration. *NEVER* leave a seriously ill patient unattended in x-ray.

5.   IVs, catheters, monitors — *assume* that something will go wrong and prepare for this ahead of time. Start with full IV bags; arrange to be notified *before* the IV runs dry... *Do not* send patients on cardiac monitors unless they are accompanied by appropriately trained personnel.

> **REMEMBER — "Dr. Murphy" is alive and well everywhere we go!**

6.   Patient's valuables — purses and wallets containing credit cards and money should never be left behind unattended in the Emergency Department or hospital floor. These should go with the patient or to a waiting family member. *ASSUME* something *will be stolen* otherwise.

> **LET'S FACE IT — No one really wants to deal with the paperwork if something gets stolen...**

RADIOGRAPHIC DECISION-MAKING — IS THERE A METHOD TO OUR MADNESS?

Though much of this information relates to primary care and emergency practice, these principles are valuable in just about *any* clinical setting.

1.   Factors affecting the decision to order an x-ray (XR):

   - Physician training and experience — specialists tend to order more x-rays (XRs) than generalists; as a physician gains experience, the frequency of ordering diagnostic x-rays decreases relative to earlier practices.

- Screening — some consider the chest x-ray (CXR) to be "routine." In the emergency department (ED) a physician may order such a film because it might give an indication that further, more complicated tests are worthwhile.

> **REMEMBER — Third party payors may not agree on the need for *routine* films!**

- Medicolegal — the percentage of x-rays ordered solely for this purpose ranges from 10-46%. The yield on these "CYA" x-rays tends to be significantly lower than those based on clinical judgement.

> ***DID YOU KNOW*** **— "CYA" really stands for "can't you analyze?"**

- Efficient time management — emergency physicians may order an x-ray before completing a history and physical examination to free themselves to see other patients.

- Reassurance — in one study, up to 30% of x-rays were done only to reassure the patient.

- Patient demands — many people insist on x-rays for "complete evaluation." Additionally, patients (and some physicians) may think an x-ray is necessary for remuneration in worker's compensation injuries and motor vehicle accidents. At times (for example, back pain), x-rays actually makes the issues *more* confusing.

- Fear of uncertainty — emergency physicians may fear mislabeling as being well patients who may have occult pathology of unknown clinical significance.

2. How to increase utility of x-ray:

- Improved history and physical examination.

- Eliminate unnecessary additional views; for example, patients under 40 years of age without suspected chest pathology do not need both a posterior-anterior *and* a lateral CXR.

- Patient education — establish rapport with patients; thoroughly explain the limitations of distinguishing abnormal from normal on x-rays.

- Increased involvement of the radiologist and radiographer — use *both* as consultants.

- Clinical audit.

- Use alternative studies — for example, ultrasound examination of the right upper quadrant is a reasonable alternative to abdominal x-ray for evaluation of cholecystitis.

X-RAY TRIAGE — A GREAT TIMESAVER...

1. Emergency department triage of single extremity trauma — data indicate excellent agreement between nursing triage and physician x-ray orders (Ropp, L., et.al., Radiograph Ordering: Agreement Between the Triage Nurse and the Physician in a Pediatric Emergency Department, Jour Emerg Med, Vol 8, 1990:697-700). For other studies (chest, abdomen, skull), there was far less agreement.

2.   Radiologic triage of the multiple trauma victim; basic portable films:

- Lateral cervical spine

- Chest x-ray (upright if possible)

- Pelvis (AP view)

3.   In-hospital triage — include during "codes," after ET tube or central line placement; some institutions have routine standing orders covering these procedures.

MEDICAL-LEGAL ASPECTS OF X-RAYS — HOW TO AVOID THE THRILL OF A SUMMONS AND THE AGONY OF A DEPOSITION!

1.   The "universal disclaimer": x-rays only show the bones. Sometimes fractures don't show; sometimes we miss seeing fractures that *are* present. You can still have a significant injury despite the presence of a "normal" x-ray.

> *REMEMBER* — A normal x-ray doesn't mean a normal patient!

2.   Patient instruction sheets — should include the policy for re-reads and missed findings, such as:

> "If you had x-rays taken at night or during the weekend, the emergency physician will make an emergency interpretation of your films; however, these films will be read again by the radiologist, usually the next day. If a discrepancy is found between the interpretation of the two doctors, you and/or your doctor will be promptly notified."

3. Emergency department follow-up of missed x-ray findings — must have a specific policy (coordinated with Radiology) to follow these up.

4. In-hospital follow-up of "routine x-rays" — if you order a film, be sure that it's read on a timely basis by a qualified individual. There must also be a means by which abnormal findings are rapidly communicated to the responsible clinician.

    > **REMEMBER — If you order the film, you're responsible for making certain that it gets appropriately read in a timely manner!**

5. Easily missed fractures: ribs, navicular, tarsal/metatarsal stress fractures.

Section 6:

Additional Reading

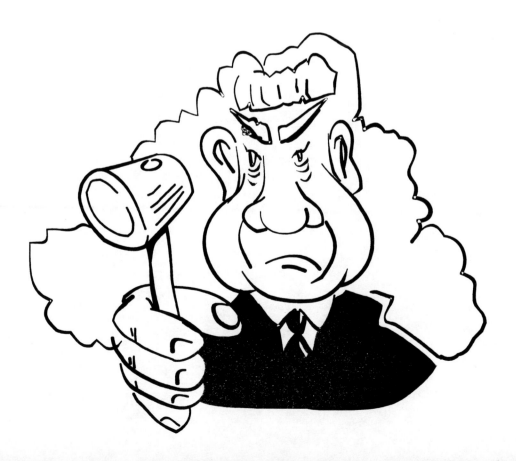

ADDITIONAL READING

Berquist, T.H., ed.; Imaging of Orthopedic Trauma and Surgery, Philadelphia, W.B. Saunders Co., 1986.

Cosgriff, H. and Anderson, D.L.; The Practice of Emergency Nursing, Philadelphia, J.B. Lippincott, 1975.

Cowley, R.A. and Dunham, C.M., eds.; Shock Trauma/Critical Care Manual, Initial Assessment and Management, Baltimore, University Park Press, 1982.

Dalinka, M.K., ed.; Emergency Medicine Clinics of North America, "Emergency Department Radiology," Philadelphia, W.B. Saunders Company, August, 1985.

Dalinka, M.K. and Kaye, J.K.; Clinics in Emergency Medicine, "Radiology in Emergency Medicine," Vol. 3, New York, Churchill Livingstone, 1984.

Felson, M., et.al.; Principles of Chest Radiology: A Programmed Text, Philadelphia, W.B. Saunders Co., 1965.

Goodman, L.R. and Putman, C.E.; Intensive Care Radiology: Imaging of the Critically Ill, Philadelphia, W.B. Saunders Co., 1983.

Hagler, M.J.; The Pocket Rad Tech, Philadelphia; W.B. Saunders Co.,1993.

Harris, J.H. and Harris, W.H.; The Radiology of Emergency Medicine, Baltimore, Williams & Wilkins Co., 1975.

Keats, T.E.; Emergency Radiology 2nd Edition, Chicago, Year Book Medical Publishers, 1989.

Levy, R.C., et.al.; Radiology in Emergency Medicine, St. Louis, C.V. Mosby Company, 1986.

Mirvis, S.E. and Young, J.W.R.; Imaging in Trauma and Critical Care, Baltimore, Williams & Wilkins Co., 1992.

Palmer, P.E.S., et.al.; WHO Basic Radiological System, Manual of Radiographic Interpretation for General Practitioners, Geneva, World Health Organization Publications, 1985.

Riddervold, H.O.; Easily Missed Fractures and Corner Signs in Radiology, Mt. Kisco, NY, Futura Publishing, 1991.

Rosen, P., et.al.; Diagnostic Radiology in Emergency Medicine, St. Louis, Mosby-Year Book, 1992.

Sproul, C. and Mullanney, P.; Emergency Care, St Louis, The CV Mosby Co., 1974.

Squires, L.F. and Novelline, R.A.; Fundamentals of Roentgenology, Cambridge, Harvard Univ. Press, 1988.

Sutton, D. and Young, J.W.R.; A Short Textbook of Clinical Imaging, London, Springer-Verlag, 1990.

Index

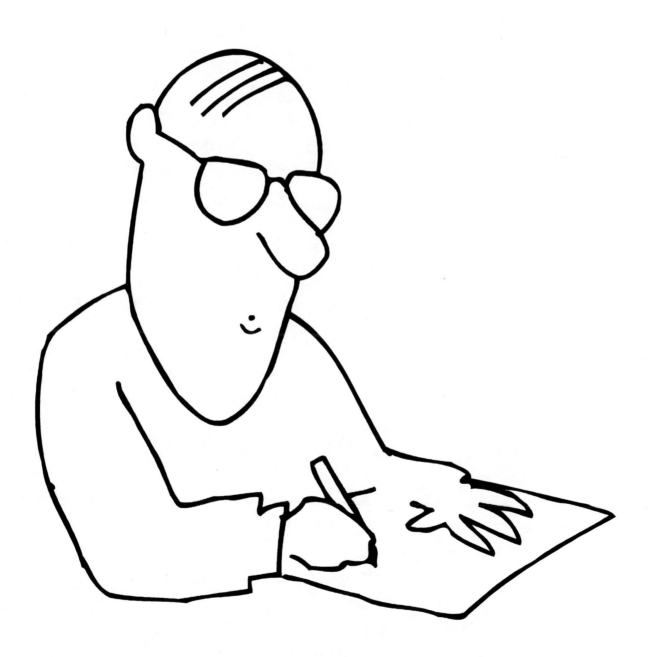

INDEX

KEY TO CHAPTERS

A = Abdomen
B = Bones
BA = Basics
C = Chest
I = Introduction
M = More Fun

Aortic aneurysm
  Abdominal   A-17
  Thoracic (traumatic)   A-17, C-1,
C-2, C-49, C-50, M-2
Abdominal CT scan   A-7, A-15
Acromioclavicular (AC) joint,
separation   B-38
Ankle joint   B-56
  Ankle mortise   B-54, B-56, B-57
  Calf tenderness, significance of in
a sprain   B-54, B-57, B-62
  Hypereversion sprain   B-57
  Hyperinversion sprain   B-54, B-
57
  Lateral malleolus   B-54
  Peroneus brevis tendon avulsion
B-54, B-62
Appendicolith   A-14
ARDS (adult respiratory distress
syndrome)   C-47, C-67

Ascites   A-11, BA-7
Asthma   C-1, C-2, C-22, C-25, C-
26
Atelectasis   C-35
Back pain   B-13, B-25, M-5
"BILL"   A-5, C-17, C-39
Border   B-35, B-36, BA-5, BA-6,
BA-8, BA-13, C-17, C-21, C-30,
C-34,   C-38-40, C-58
Calcaneal fractures   B-57, B-62
  Boehler's angle in calcaneal
fractures   B-58, B-59
Cardiac shadow (see also cardiac
silhouette, heart shadow)   C-8, C-
58
Cardiac silhouette (see also
cardiac shadow, heart shadow)   C-
4, C-8
Carina   C-54, C-55, C-69
Central venous pressure

monitoring lines C-56

Chest tree C-1, C-3

Chest tubes C-55

Chronic obstructive pulmonary disease (COPD) C-9, C-25

Clavicle fractures B-38

Clinical diagnosis C-41, C-47, C-67

Coin lesions on chest x-ray (see also "masses") C-60

Colle's fracture B-34

Congestive heart failure C-1, C-2, C-42, C-45, C-46, C-48
  Cephalization of flow C-44, C-45
    Deer antlers C-45
    Kerley lines C-45
    Pulmonary edema ("snowball appearance") C-45

COPD (chronic obstructive pulmonary disease) C-1, C-2, C-9, C-10, C-25, C-26, C-66
  Cor pulmonale C-25, C-44

Coracoclavicular ligament B-39

Costophrenic angles C-1, C-7, C-8, C-37, C-63

Degenerative osteoarthritis B-13
  Arthritic spurs B-13
  Osteophytes B-13

Diaphragm shadows A-4, C-1, C-4, C-6
  Paper-thin diaphragm A-17, C-23

Elbow joint B-35-38, B-61
  Anterior fat pad B-35, B-37, B-61
  Fat pad sign B-37
  Posterior fat pad B-36, B-37, B-61

Empyema C-28

Facial bones B-1, B-8

Femur fractures B-50, B-62

Flank fat stripes A-4

Foot B-1, B-2, BA-10, B-54, B-56, B-57, B-59, C-51

Foreign bodies A-1, A-12, A-13, B-8, C-2, C-61

Free (intraperitoneal) air A-1, A-4-7, A-17, C-7
  Paper-thin diaphragm A-17, C-23

Gallstones A-14

Goodpasture's syndrome C-42

Greenstick fracture B-4

Heart shadow (see also cardiac shadow, cardiac silhouette) C-8-10, C-13, C-25, C-31, C-34, C-45

Heart BA-6, BA-7, BA-9, BA-10, C-1, C-2, C-8-11, C-13, C-14, C-21, C-22, C-25, C-30, C-31, C-34, C-38-40, C-42-48, C-56, C-58, C-59, C-66, C-67
  Hypertrophy C-8, C-43, C-44
  Hypoplasia C-8
  Left ventricle C-8, C-42, C-59
  Pulmonary artery C-10, C-57, C-58, C-69
  Right atrium C-56, C-58
  Right ventricle C-8, C-42, C-58, C-59

Hemidiaphragm C-6, C-7, C-13, C-63

Hemithorax C-7, C-19, C-23, C-28, C-31, C-32, C-40

Hilar markings C-1, C-10, C-11

Hip B-43

  Hip dislocations B-43, B-47, B-48, B-62

  Hip fractures B-48, BA-12

Infiltrates BA-7, C-1, C-4, C-5, C-12, C-27, C-35, C-38, C-39, C-42, C-46, C-47, C-67

  Infiltrates, alveolar C-35

  Infiltrates, interstitial C-35

  Infiltrates, plate-like C-35

  Infiltrates, streaky C-35

Inspiration C-4, C-5, C-61

Interface A-5, BA-5, BA-6, BA-13, C-6, C-20, C-21, C-33, C-38, C-39

Knee joint B-50, B-51

Lag time C-48

Lunate dislocation B-32, B-33

Lung, lobar anatomy C-38

  Lingula C-38, C-39

  Lower lobes C-39, C-40

  Middle lobe C-38, C-39

  Upper lobes C-11, C-38, C-39, C-44

Lung markings C-1, C-11, C-12, C-14, C-15, C-19-21, C-24, C-31, C-33, C-34, C-37, C-46, C-63, C-64

Mandible fractures B-10

Masses on chest x-ray, potential

causes B-8, C-2, C-5, C-59

  Osteoblastic lesions C-53

  Sarcoidosis C-61

Maxillary fractures B-10

Medical-legal aspects of x-rays M-1, M-7

Metacarpals B-25

Missed fractures (easily missed) C-51, M-8

  Navicular bone of the wrist I-8

  Rib fractures C-1, C-49, C-51, C-52

Motility disturbances A-1, A-4, A-10

  Bowel obstruction A-7

  Ileus A-7, A-8

  Springs A-9, A-10, A-17

  Tunnels A-9, A-10, A-17

  Turtle shells A-9

Nasogastric tubes A-12

Navicular bone of the wrist I-8

Nipple shadows BA-11, C-53

Noncardiogenic pulmonary edema (ARDS) C-1, C-47

Orbital blow-out fracture B-8

Osteoblastic lesions C-53

Osteolytic lesions C-53

Osteoporosis B-11, B-12, C-52

Over-penetrated x-ray C-5

Pancreatitis A-13

Patella B-29, B-51

Pelvis A-2, B-1, B-2, B-45, B-50, B-62 BA-12, BA-13, C-53, M-7

Penetration C-4, C-5

Pericardial effusion C-1, C-8, C-

34

Perilunate dislocation B-32

Phalanges, significance of associated soft tissue injuries B-25, B-59

Collateral ligaments B-26, B-27, B-50

Extensor tendons B-26, B-27

Volar plates B-26, B-27

Pleural effusion B-38, C-1, C-7, C-8, C-27-31, C-33, C-34, C-48-50, C-56, C-65, C-67, C-69

Loculated pleural effusion C-27

Meniscus (fluid level) C-28, C-31, C-32

Posterior costophrenic angle C-29

Posterior sulcus C-29, C-30, C-67

Pneumomediastinum C-22, C-26, C-66

Pneumonia C-1, C-2, C-37, C-40, C-41, C-47-49, C-66, I-7, I-8

Pneumocystis carinii pneumonia C-41

Pneumoperitoneum A-5

Pneumothorax B-38, BA-11, C-1, C-16, C-17, C-19-22, C-26, C-46, C-51, C-52, C-56, C-66, C-69, M-2

Pneumothorax, tension C-21

Prevertebral space swelling B-20

Primary survey BA-8

Psoas muscle shadows A-2, A-4

Pulmonary artery flow-directed catheters (Swan-Ganz) C-57

Pulmonary contusion C-1, C-2, C-42, C-48, C-49, C-52, C-67

Pulmonary embolism, with and without infarction C-1, C-48

Pulmonary hyperinflation C-10

Radiodense BA-3, BA-4, C-17

Radiographer B-21, B-41, I-1, I-5, I-6, M-1, M-2, M-6

Radiologic technologist I-5

Radiological density BA-3

Radiolucent B-4, B-8 B-35, B-53, BA-1-5, BA-10, BA-12, C-7, C-9, C-17, C-22, C-34

Radiopaque A-12, A-14, B-3, B-8, B-24, BA-1-5, BA-7, BA-8, BA-10, BA-12, C-13, C-17, C-19, C-23, C-24, C-26, C-33, C-34, C-46, C-53, C-55, C-56, C-58-62

Requisitions M-1

Retropharyngeal abscess B-17

Rib fractures C-1, C-49, C-51, C-52

Roentgen BA-1, BA-2

Rotation B-43, B-47, B-62, C-4, C-5

Rules of the spine B-11

Rupture of the diaphragm C-2, C-23, C-66

Sarcoidosis C-61

Secondary survey BA-8

Sesamoid bones B-29

Shoulder joint B-42, B-62

Dislocation   B-48, B-62

Sinusitis   B-2

Skull fracture   B-2, B-8

Depressed skull fracture   B-2

Suture line   B-5, B-6

Vascular markings, normal   B-2

Sternoclavicular joint   B-38

Subluxation   B-14

Tibial plateau   B-51

Tibial plateau, fractures   B-53

Vertebral bodies   B-11-17, B-20-22, B-25, C-3, C-5

Vertebral compression fracture B-2

Vertebral interspaces   C-3

**Thanks
so
much
for
using
this
book. I
hope
you had
as
much
fun
reading
it as I did writing it... Mikel**

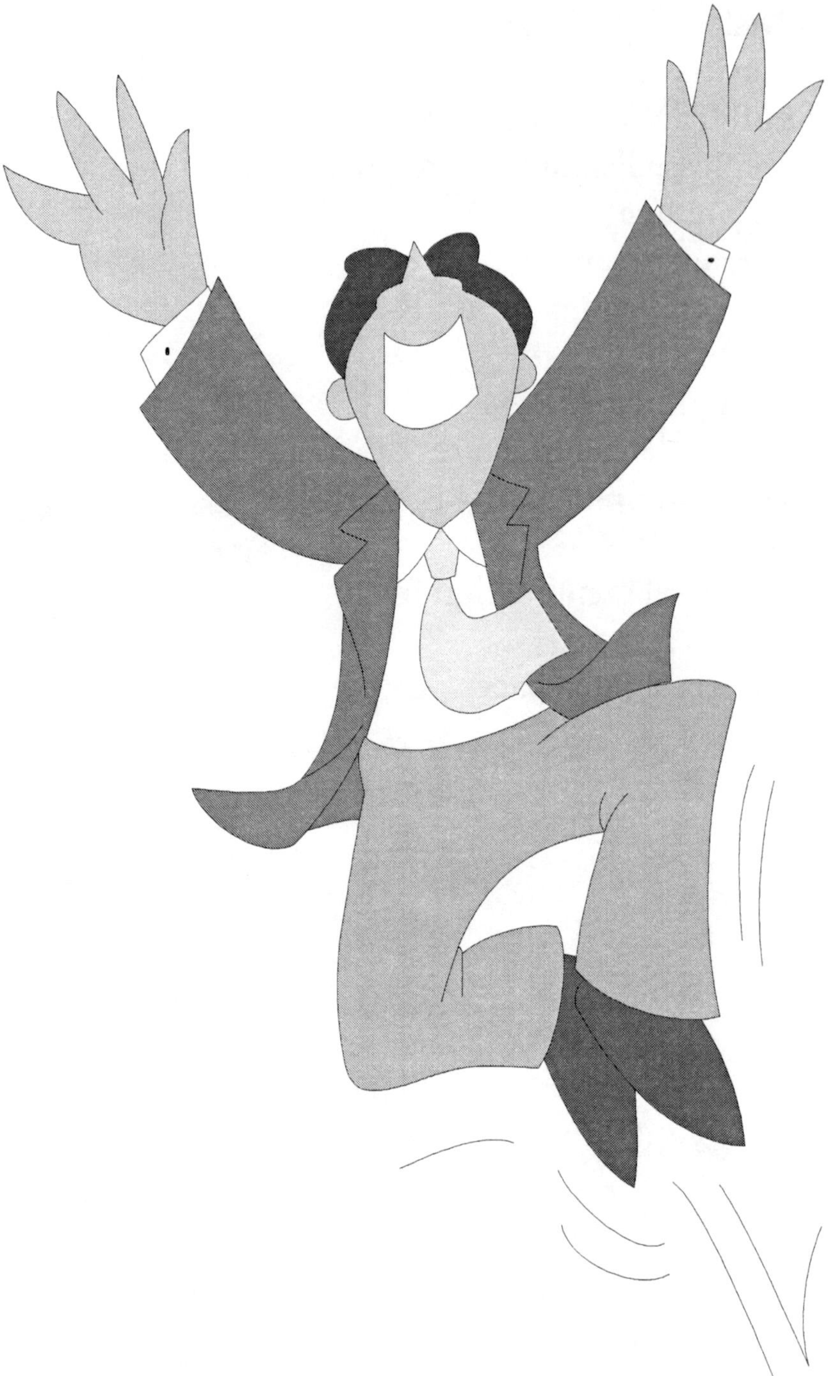

TAKE A FRESH APPROACH TO IN-HOUSE CONTINUING EDUCATION

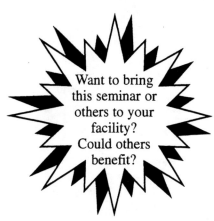

Want to bring this seminar or others to your facility? Could others benefit?

WE BRING IT TO YOU

PESI HealthCare has invested a lot of resources into each program, with the constant intention of improvement. All programs have been presented many times in the public arena and feedback has been utilized to improve each and every seminar, including outline, written materials and speaker's presentation. Excellent bound written materials, designed to reduce note-taking are included for each attendee. These are not a small pile of handouts in a folder. You will receive valuable, current research, charts, interventions etc. All courses are approved for continuing education credits and PESI HealthCare will take care of continuing education administration and recordkeeping. Let us remove the hassle of program development and execution for you. From clinical to management programs, give us a call today!

HERES THE DEAL . . .

We provide:
- Curriculum design
- Honorarium to faculty
- Printing and shipping of bound written materials to your location
- All contact hour accreditation administration, including certificates and 7-year record-keeping
- Tips and techniques for successful on-site facilitation
- Graphic design assistance for promotional brochures (optional)

Your organization provides:
- Meeting facility
- Faculty travel and lodging

FLEXIBLE PRICING*

Our pricing is structured to allow for a necessary minimum fee, with a sliding scale that allows for price drops as attendee numbers increase. If you desire to promote outside your organization, that is fine, and you can price tuition at whatever level you desire.

$2000 minimum for first 25 people
$45 per person for the next 26-45 people
$40 per person for the next 46- 75 people
For more than 75 people, call for pricing

These prices are to be used as guidelines only and will vary based on length of program, faculty and other variables. Pricing is subject to change, please call for specific pricing.

subject to change

A WIDE SELECTION OF PROGRAM TOPICS INCLUDE:

- Geriatric Problem Assessment & Emergencies
- Cardiac Emergencies
- Critical Care Update
- Infectious Diseases- Into the Millennium
- Competency
- Psychiatric Emergencies
- Managing the Med/Surg Client
- Understanding Laboratory Tests
- Respiratory Emergencies
- Essential Physical Assessment Skills
- Critical Thinking Skills
- Understanding X-rays: A Plain English Approach
- Pharmacology
- Geriatric Pharmacology
- Pediatric Emergencies
- Mental Health Problems in the Elderly
- Hemodynamic Monitoring
- Nursing and the Law
- Supervisory Management
- Case Management
- Telephone Triage: How to Practice Nursing Over the Phone
- Organ Failure
- Geriatric Problem Assessment
- Common Medical Emergencies
- Plain English Pathophysiology
- Sentinel Events
- Medication Errors
- Risk Management for Hospitals
- 12-Lead EKG Made Easy
- Neurological Emergencies
- Skin and Wound Caring
- Your Amazing Brain
- Herbs in Healthcare
- Managing Heart Failure
- And more

call us today!!

800-472-6930
Ask for Patti Johnson

Visit our website at:
www.pesihealthcare.com/contract.htm

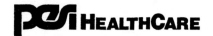